What other Physicians are saying about Passing on Bypass

"In language as compelling as the importance of the subject matter, Dr. Juetersonke reveals well-guarded secrets about coronary heart disease, its usual treatment and important options such as ECP. Unless *Passing on Bypass* becomes required reading for all cardiology fellows and practitioners, it may represent the best "second opinion" anyone (faced with angina or a failed treadmill test) can obtain. Courageously written, this book could easily save thousands from making an unnecessary journey to cardiac surgery."

James Ehrlich, MD
Medical Director, Colorado Heart Imaging
Medical Co-Director, HeartScan Houston
and HeartScan Washington DC

"Dr. Juetersonke has performed a great service for all of us, as *Passing on Bypass* presents an excellent critique of modern invasive cardiology using up-to-date references from the best available conventional medicine and cardiology journals. This is followed by an FDA-cleared, non-invasive, safe and effective alternative for coronary artery disease called external counterpulsation or ECP. It should be read by all health care professionals and anyone concerned about his/her heart—especially those people with coronary artery disease and angina pectoris. I supplied my whole clinical staff with copies and recommend it daily to my cardiac patients."

Michael B.

"My own personal e
with EECP® has been 100%
truly remarkable."

Nancy R. Cho, MD FACC
Director of the Advanced Cardiac
Treatment Center

"We have been involved in the delivery of EECP® service for nearly two years. Our experience has been that a vast majority of patients feel that this procedure substantially improves their quality of life as well as reducing or eliminating chest pain. The combination of minimal risk and profound improvement makes this a desirable procedure in the mind of most patients and many physicians. We salute your effort to bring this important and potentially life saving information to the public."

Michael E. Eads MD,
VP HeartGen Centers, Inc.

Fix your heart without surgery!
You can join the smart people who are...

Passing On Bypass

Using External CounterPulsation:
An FDA Cleared Alternative To
Treat Heart Disease Without
Surgery, Drugs Or Angioplasty!

Dedication

To my parents and family who gave me the opportunity, to my wife Sandy and my daughter Lora for their love and support which made this book possible and to my patients who have taught me much.

In memory of Hans E. Juetersonke and Carol A. Klassen.

Acknowledgements

Barry Weiner, for his exceptional ability and patience in getting this published.

Lynn Boutte for my photograph.

George Zirfas and James Rutz for the cover design.

Jewel Shanahan for her help.

My staff, family, friends, physicians, patients and the many others who helped make this book possible.

Table of Contents

Table of Contents

Foreward

Dear Reader:

My name is Dr. George J. Juetersonke and I am a physician in Colorado Springs. Sometimes my patients have a hard time saying my name (jew-ter-son-key), so they just call me "Dr. J." If you, or a friend, or loved one has heart disease then this book is for you. Despite all the major advances in medicine, heart disease is still the number one killer of both men and women. In the pages that follow you will have the opportunity to learn about a revolutionary new treatment that could dramatically improve the quality of your life or that of a loved one.

For the past twenty years I have focused my medical practice on helping the "hard to treat patient." By hard to treat, I refer to patients who have lost confidence in today's impersonal and confusing health-care environment. It's no secret that most managed care providers simply don't want to deal with people who are chronically ill.

Such indifference can be a real problem for people with coronary heart disease and the debilitating fatigue, chest pressure, and shortness of breath often associated with it. Of course people with heart difficulties can't simply ignore their condition-that could be fatal.

Given this rather sorry situation, I needed to find a simpler, safer, less expensive treatment for my heart patients. I'm pleased to report that my research led me to a new, FDA-cleared treatment that holds terrific promise for coronary patients who suffer with angina (chest pain) and wish to avoid bypass surgery and angioplasty.

My medical colleagues call this new treatment External CounterPulsation or ECP (sometimes also referred to as enhanced external counterpulsation). In my office we call this exciting new treatment *LifePULSE®*. It uses a simple process that allows the heart's own rhythm to circulate blood back to the heart muscle when it is resting (called diastole). This treatment literally encourages the heart to grow its own bypasses around blockages naturally, without surgery or drugs! Many insurances and Medicare will often pay a portion of the costs in selected cases.

My philosophy about medicine is that patients who are the best informed about their treatment options and work as partners with their Healthcare professionals receive better care than people who simply defer all their decisions to their doctor. In that spirit, I hope you will read this book and if you know of someone that might benefit from learning about this innovative treatment then please pass this book on to him or her.

If you have Internet access, you may also want to visit my *LifePULSE®* web site at: www.drjlifepulse.com

This site is proving to be very helpful to those seeking an alternative to bypass surgery and/or angioplasty. It has a really good presentation of the procedure and its benefits. If you require even more in-depth information, we offer a number of hot links to other sites, including the American Heart Association, where you can read up on the latest studies and scientific data.

Find out if *LifePULSE®* ECP is the right choice for you or that loved one with heart disease. It may just be that *LifePULSE®* ECP will be the answer that you have been searching for.

Best wishes for a heart healthy future,
George J. Juetersonke, D.O.

Remember that *LifePULSE®* External CounterPulsation is FDA cleared and eligible for insurance as well as Medicare reimbursement.

Say Good-bye to Heart Surgery

It had to happen! After decades of subjecting heart patients to painful and dangerous surgical procedures, a non-surgical, drug-free treatment is finally available. What I have to tell you may surprise you. It is perhaps the best-kept secret in modern American medicine! The information I will present to you could save you or a loved one untold suffering and maybe even your life. I have spent the last 24 years searching for alternatives to coronary artery bypass surgery (known as coronary artery bypass graft or CABG pronounced 'CABBAGE') and angioplasty (known as PTCA or percutaneous transluminal coronary angioplasty). What I have found could dramatically change your future for the better.

Imagine a not too distant future when we will look at bypass surgery, stents, and angioplasty as the obsolete, dangerous and expensive procedures that they are.

A new way has now been found that does not use surgery to treat heart disease and its biggest symptom, angina. For the first time since the invention of heart surgery a program has been designed to treat angina using the body's own ability to heal itself! The latest in computer microprocessors, mechanical and electric engineering, physics and an in-depth understanding of the physiology of the coronary circulatory system has been combined by scientists to develop a treatment that encourages the heart to heal itself. This new technology, called External CounterPulsation is so safe and simple it is amazing it wasn't thought of sooner. ECP* is a noninvasive procedure that allows patients to grow their own bypasses naturally. It often works even in cases where bypass surgery or angioplasty has failed or wasn't completely successful.

ECP is so effective it will change what PTCA stands for. In the future PTCA will stand for *Put That Catheter Away* and CABG will stand for *Can Avoid Bypass Grafting!*

Why haven't you heard more about it? Let me explain. It does seem hard at first to comprehend the reluctance that hospitals, doctors and insurance companies have in accepting such a safe, simple, affordable and effective therapy. That is until one realizes that coronary artery bypass surgery has become a multi-billion-dollar industry! Eugene Braunwald, M.D., foresaw this potential as early as 1977 when his editorial was published in the *New England Journal of Medicine*. Dr. Braunwald stated: "An even more insidious problem is that what might be considered an 'industry' is being built around this operation..."

For a more recent perspective, one only needs to look at the use of stents for coronary artery disease. (Stents are small expandable springs that are surgically placed inside the coronary arteries in order to prop open blockages.) In the December 1998 issue of the *New England Journal of Medicine*, Eric J. Topol, M.D. from the renown Cleveland Clinic writes that in 1994 there were essentially zero stent placements in the United States. Within three years the number of stents placed went from zero to over 800,000 and is now a 1.5 billion dollar industry! Dr. Topol reports that the profit margin per stent is between 85 to 95% with the average cost of a stent in this country at $1,500. (In Canada the same stent is only $650.) This illustrates how quickly both bypass surgery and its counterpart stent surgery have been marketed into industries almost overnight.

Stents have only been used for about five years. Contrast this with ECP, which has almost 47 years of research behind it. Ask your doctor what will happen to implanted stents in ten or twenty years from now? Will we have another silicone fiasco? Nobody knows for sure. Yet the average heart patient receives almost two stents. Do you feel comfortable having one of these objects placed in your chest for the rest of your life? Did you know that they cannot be taken out once placed in a coronary artery?

In fact the latest research from Mount Sinai Hospital, University of Toronto, Canada shows that this may indeed be a previously unrecognized problem! Paul R.A. Caramori, M.D. and colleagues examined thirty-nine patients that had a stent, angioplasty or arthrectomy for blockages of the left coronary artery. Several months after the procedure only the patients that had a stent placed showed significant inflammation and dysfunction of the lining of the blood vessel. Gregory D. Tilton, M.D. states in an accompanying editorial in the *Journal of the American College of Cardiology* that this new research sounds a warning that there exists the potential for long-term adverse complications from stent placement. Obviously further study is needed.

To make matters worse it has been shown in many cases that surgery, stents and angioplasty do not prolong life, that the recommended surgery is often unnecessary and that repeat surgery is frequently required to maintain improvement. Don't we all know someone who has had to have repeat surgery for coronary heart disease? If I were to buy a lottery ticket in Colorado my chances of winning are one in a million. But if I were to bet on your chances of dying, suffering a heart attack or having angina within the first year after bypass surgery or angioplasty, my chances of being correct could be as high as two out of ten! Does this sound like success?

What about the odds of a younger person with a heart attack being able to get back to work? Which has a better chance of getting you back to work: surgery, angioplasty, or medical treatment without surgery? Duke University researchers found that after one year the chances of a heart patient being back to work were 8 out of 10, regardless of whether they had surgery or medical treatment without surgery. Not a very strong endorsement for angioplasty or bypass, is it? The point is that even though stents and surgery do not work that well for the patient, they work very well for the cardiac industry's bottom line! What incentive is there to change when you have a monopoly on the only treatment of heart disease, the nation's number one killer?

Is it any wonder then that you and your physician have not heard about this exciting new treatment that threatens a whole multi-billion dollar industry? How do you and your physicians fight the medical equivalent of Microsoft®? People with life yet to live continue to undergo expensive, dangerous surgical treatments that do not necessarily prolong life. That is why I felt it necessary to write this book. Armed with the information in this book you will be able to make a truly informed decision about *all* the options available for treating heart disease.

There are alternatives and this is one you should know about.

Here comes the good part, imagine:

- No surgical scars

- No grafts taken from your leg, no 12-inch scars on your legs

- No anesthesia

- No catheters threaded through your groin

- No x-ray exposure or risk of radiation burns

- No hospital gowns or hospital stays

- No distraught loved ones

- No worry about surviving the procedure

- No stay in intensive care, no ventilators

- No extensive period of rehabilitation

- No brain injury from being on a heart lung machine

Now read about this technological breakthrough.

External CounterPulsation* for coronary heart disease and angina is:

- Safe

- Simple

- Elegant, noninvasive

- Affordable (a fraction of the cost compared to surgery or angioplasty)

- Works for a wide variety of patients

- FDA cleared for angina

- Enables your heart to grow its own bypasses naturally without surgery or drugs and is conveniently performed in your doctor's office

- Covered by most insurances**

- Medicare covered.***

In the pages that follow, you will learn about a treatment that takes only 35 hours (one hour a day, five days a week, for seven weeks.) While receiving these treatments, you lay comfortably on a padded table and can take a nap, listen to music or talk to your spouse or friend.

You now have a choice

Don't stop here

Find out what the heart surgery industry doesn't want you to know

L   Life, start living and enjoying life
I   Incredible, innovative therapy, insurance covered
F   For anyone young or old
E   Exciting new discovery

P   Proven results
U   Unique therapy for those unwilling or unable to have surgery
L   Love treatment, you will feel so much healthier
S   Safe and simple
E   Easy and effective

*Please note that there are several terms that are often used: CardiAssist™ CounterPulsation System, which is a trademark of Cardiomedics, or enhanced external counterpulsation, EECP® which is a trademark of Vasomedical, or double E-CP. Other abbreviations used include ECP, SECP, and EC. For the purposes of this book the generic abbreviation ECP will be used for both External CounterPulsation and Enhanced External CounterPulsation.

**However, since it is so new, you might have to educate your insurance carrier about External CounterPulsation.

***Medicare covered for patients with inoperable Canadian Classification Stage 3 or 4 angina. Stage 4 is the most severe kind of angina one can have. This is subject to change.

References:
Braunwald E. Coronary-artery surgery at the crossroads. N Eng J Med Sep 22;297(12):661-663.

Topol EJ. Coronary-artery-stents--gauging, gorging, and gouging. N. Eng J Med 1998 Dec 3;339(23):1702-1704.

Tilton GD. Can stents damage coronary arteries remote from the stent? J Am Coll Cardiol 1999 Nov 15; 34(6):1680-1681.

Caramori PR, Lima VC, Seidelin PH, et al. Long-term endothelial dysfunction after coronary artery stenting. J Am Coll Cardiol 1999 Nov 15;34(6):1675-1679.

Chapter 1
What's Wrong With the Way We Treat Heart Disease?

Since 1920, coronary heart disease has been the number one killer in the United States. Over 58 million Americans have some kind of heart disease. The American Heart Association estimates that every thirty seconds an American will suffer a coronary event and that every minute someone will die from a myocardial infarction commonly known as a heart attack. It is estimated that in the last twelve months alone, over one million one hundred thousand Americans will have had their first or second heart attack. The breakdown is as follows: for 650,000 of these people it will be their first heart attack, 450,000 will be having their second heart attack. About one third of the people experiencing these heart attacks will die from them. This is not to be thought of as a disease that affects mostly men! Figures show that more than half a million women die from cardiovascular disease each year. This is more than all forms of cancer combined!

The average cost of cardiac catheterization in the United States in 1998 was approximately $20,000 with over two million procedures being performed. This is an increase of almost 350% from 1979. Researchers predict that by the year 2010 there will be over 3 million cardiac catheterizations performed annually.

According to the American Heart Association, the number of coronary bypass surgeries is also increasing rapidly. About 230% more coronary artery bypasses were done last year than in 1979. It is estimated that in 1996 there were 600,000 coronary artery bypass surgeries performed. The estimated average cost of bypass surgery is approximately $60,000 to $70,000. While the United States is home to only about 5% of the entire world's population, doctors here performed almost 50% of all heart surgeries done in the entire world.

One reason for this impressive growth is the fact that coronary angiography acts as a pipeline that sends patients ultimately to angioplasty or bypass surgery. In an article in the *Journal of the American Medical Association*, Thomas B. Graboys, M.D. explains that there are many non-medical reasons for the explosive growth of invasive cardiac procedures.

First, cardiac procedures are very profitable. In fact, hospital administrators often refer to the Cardiology Department as the profit center of the hospital.

Second, we have trained too many cardiologists and in order for these cardiologists to keep up their certification they must perform a minimum number of procedures every year. Furthermore, it is a closed system, the same doctor doing the angiogram will also be the same doctor recommending and performing the angioplasty. Would a second opinion from a different doctor always agree with the need for surgery? Later on in this book you will read that second opinions often disagree with the need for surgical procedures.

Finally, patients are often unnecessarily scared into surgery when the doctor shows them the angiogram and announces; this artery is what we call a 'widow maker', it is a critical lesion, if we don't operate you will be dead by Christmas, you are a walking time bomb. You may be shocked to find out that these scare tactics are not supported by the scientific research. As you will read later, a physician cannot tell by looking at an angiogram whether a blockage will cause a heart attack or not! And just as important is the little known fact that the risk of death or heart attack is only 2% per year in patients with stable coronary artery disease. This statistic is so poorly known that most physicians, when asked what they believed the patients risk of death or heart attack to be was, gave wildly inflated estimates of 15% to 50% per year. When this 2% per year heart attack or death rate for coronary artery disease is compared with the 4% to 8% risk of death from bypass surgery, a startling fact is realized. The surgical cure for coronary artery disease can be more deadly than the disease itself.

Furthermore, Dr. Graboys questions whether cardiologists

when obtaining consent to perform an angiogram or angioplasty clearly explain the risks of stroke, heart attack, or even death as well as all the other less serious complications that may occur.

The medical journal *Lancet*, published an article known as RITA-2 (randomized intervention treatment of angina study) in 1997, in which over one thousand stable angina patients were randomly assigned to receive either medication or angioplasty. After little more than two and one half years it was found that angioplasty patients had 90% more deaths and heart attacks than those patients receiving only medical therapy. Even more significant was that the risk of death, heart attack, or coronary artery bypass surgery was 42% lower in the patients that had medical therapy instead of angioplasty! The results of this study does not provide any evidence to support the belief of many doctors that successful angioplasty of a severe coronary artery stenosis actually reduces the risk of heart attack.

As expensive as this surgery is, it is also very discouraging to know that coronary artery bypass surgery and angioplasty will rarely allow a patient to get off of their cardiac medications. Surprisingly, there is no research to prove that all patients receiving these treatments live longer. Repeat surgeries and angioplasties are all too common. Don't we all know somebody who has had to go back for an additional procedure? One journal reported that up to half of all bypass patients will require repeat surgery within ten years. It is obvious then that coronary artery bypass surgery and angioplasty do not cure heart disease! In fact, James S. Forrester, M.D. from Cedars Sinai Center in Los Angeles stated in the 1997 issue of *Circulation,* "We believe that the illusion of cardiology is that bypass or dilatation of coronary stenosis reduces the risk of myocardial infarction."

K. Lance Gould, M.D., from the University of Texas Medical School, Houston, Texas, stated in a 1998 article in the *American Journal of Medicine* that new knowledge of how coronary atherosclerosis contributes to heart disease should lead us to a new treatment protocol. In his approach to coronary heart disease, angioplasty and bypass surgery would only be used as a last resort. He states: "Noninvasive management of coronary artery disease based on reversal treatment is a valid, safe, effective primary step, but it requires patient and physician knowledge." Dr. Gould goes on to say that heart disease should be treated immediately and aggressively with a strict diet (lower saturated fat and, if indicated, lower carbohydrates), weight control, medicines to control angina, aspirin to prevent clots and statin drugs to lower cholesterol to less than 140. He concludes by explaining that only for the minority of patients not responding to aggressive medical treatment would coronary angiograms, angioplasty and coronary surgery be appropriate.

The information presented in this book is not meant to discourage anyone from seeking help for their heart disease. It is presented with the goal of informing you about the treatments available and what might be the expected outcome. If you have any doubts about the procedures that your doctor has recommended, please obtain a second opinion. It has been said that the most damaging phrase in the English language is, "We've always done it this way." The time is past due for a better, safer alternative to surgery. External CounterPulsation is changing the face of cardiology.

References:
Graboys, TB. Coronary angiography a long look at a short queue. JAMA. 1999;282:184-185.

Coronary angioplasty versus medical therapy for angina: the second Randomized Intervention Treatment of Angina (RITA-2) trial. RITA-2 trial participants. Lancet 1997 Aug 16;350(9076):461-468.

Forrester JS, Shah PK. Lipid lowering versus revascularization: an idea whose time (for testing) has come. Circulation 1997 Aug 19;96(4):1360-1362.

Gould KL. New concepts and paradigms in cardiovascular medicine: the noninvasive management of coronary artery disease. Am J Med 1999;104: 2-17.

Enas EA. Testing the efficacy of lipid-lowering therapy versus revascularization: the time has come, or is it past due? Circulation 1998 Jun 30;97(25):2584-2586.

Chapter 2

Start Living Again, True Patient Stories[*]

In 1990, 55-year-old Mike Larson went to his doctor with chest pain. An angiogram revealed that Mr. Larson had severe three-vessel disease with significant blockages. At his doctor's recommendation, Mr. Larson underwent quadruple bypass surgery using non-essential veins from his legs as bypass material. He seemed to recover well and went for seven years without any chest pain.

In 1997, Mr. Larson's angina suddenly returned and he suffered a heart attack shortly thereafter. Another angiogram revealed that all four bypass grafts had completely closed off. This time his doctor suggested angioplasty, which Mr. Larson agreed to undergo. Immediately following inflation of the angioplasty balloons, small metal coils called "stents" were inserted into Mr. Larson's grafts, and he was put on a blood thinner to discourage the clotting that often occurs within stents. Unfortunately, as is the case in about 20 percent of stent recipients, Mr. Larson improved for approximately 6 months, at which time the stents became blocked.

At this point Mr. Larson began to experience angina so severe, just getting ready for bed at night brought it on. The only way he could walk even a short distance was to take nitroglycerin; something he was forced to do up to 10 times a day. By now his only options were to repeat bypass surgery or try something else.

Desperate, his wife began a vigorous search for alternatives to surgery. By chance, she came across a pamphlet on External CounterPulsation. Although very skeptical, Mr. Larson agreed to see a physician equipped to perform this new technique in the next town. Impressed with ECP's simplicity, safety, and success record, he decided to undergo the typical regimen: one treatment per day five days per week for 7 weeks. At the end of the thirty-fifth treatment, Mr. Larson reported significantly less chest pain during short walks or moderate exertion but said he still experienced it if he walked too far or otherwise overexerted himself. A subsequent series of treatments further reduced his symptoms. To date, Mr. Larson has had 105 treatments. He can walk for an unlimited period, is totally off of nitroglycerin, and cannot remember the last time he experienced any kind of chest pain.

As is explained in Chapter 9, External CounterPulsation therapy forces fresh, oxygenated blood into the coronary arteries, encouraging expansion of the collateral vessels and oxygenation of the heart muscle itself. The procedure can also result in permanent enlargement of the collateral vessels and, even more amazing, development of collateral offshoots—brand new vessels which further aid in the delivery of fresh blood to the heart. With an adequate supply of oxygen, the heart's only means of complaining--angina--subsides.

This is precisely what appears to have happened in Mr. Larson's heart. A post-ECP angiogram revealed that the collateral blood vessels had significantly enlarged and had "sprouted" quite a few new vessels. It also showed that the original bypasses remained closed. In other words, all of the blood nourishing Mr. Larson's heart was coming from the collateral vessels and their offspring. Little to none was flowing from the bypasses! In a sense, Mr. Larson had grown his own bypasses and had done so naturally, without a single incision or puncture.

Mr. Larson continues to receive periodic "booster" ECP treatments. He also exercises on a regular basis, something angina prevented him from doing even moderately before ECP and something that itself contributes to the daily oxygenation and well-being of Mr. Larson's heart.

In addition to ECP, Mr. Larson's doctor prescribed a special diet, omega-3 essential fats, and Lipitor™ (Parke-Davis), also known as atorvastatin. Since taking up this cholesterol-fighting regimen, Mr.

Larson's cholesterol is down from 250 to 150, and his triglycerides are down from 500 into the 100s.

As a result of External CounterPulsation, Mr. Larson should be able to live a longer, healthier life. Fortunately, he found out about it prior to undergoing more bypass surgery.

Kevin Schatz

Kevin Schatz first experienced angina 19 years ago while shoveling his home out of a thick Michigan snow. The pain was sudden and severe, radiating all the way from his heart to his jaw. When an angiogram revealed advanced three-vessel disease, his doctor scheduled Mr. Schatz for immediate triple-bypass surgery.

Instead of giving in, as most patients in such high-pressured situations do, the 55-year-old Ford Aerospace engineer began asking questions. Was surgery his only hope for survival? Must he risk his life to save it? Or were less radical options available? On the advice of another physician, Mr. Schatz declined surgery and elected to go on the low-fat Pritikin diet.

The choice turned out to be a good one. Mr. Schatz lived 15 years before the pain returned, this time with more frequency and under less stressful conditions such as when he was walking or eating. It wasn't long before a stroll around the house brought on an episode of angina and the 69-year-old feared such common endeavors as climbing the stairs or planting a shrub.

Still leery of surgery, Mr. Schatz searched for alternatives and even tried 40 treatments of chelation therapy: the intravenous infusion of a synthetic amino acid called ethylene-diamine-tetra-acetic acid (EDTA) which has been reported to relieve angina in some patients. While chelation therapy has precluded surgery for many, it only provided limited relief for Mr. Schatz. His angina persisted and discouragement set in.

Were bypass surgery and angioplasty his only remaining options? He shuddered at the thought of having to undergo a surgical procedure that might leave him in worse shape than he was in. After all, there were no guarantees that heart surgery would fix his condition. Even if it did, the "fix" would most likely be temporary and could even accelerate the need for a second bypass surgery.

Mr. Schatz expanded his search for alternatives to the Internet where, at last, he came upon information on the existence of External CounterPulsation therapy. Mr. Schatz was fortunate enough to find a doctor in his area who was familiar with the procedure and scheduled an appointment to see him. The doctor performed an electrocardiogram which revealed decreased blood flow to the heart, even when Mr. Schatz was resting.

Thirty-five ECP treatments later, Mr. Schatz felt like a new man. His electrocardiogram is normal, and he is virtually angina-free, taking nitroglycerin only on rare occasions. The man who could not plant a single shrub recently planted 24 without difficulty. He can also climb stairs—twelve flights of them, to be exact—without stopping.

Mr. Schatz is scheduled to undergo another 35 treatments on the counterpulsation unit. After completing these, it is anticipated that he will need no heart medication whatsoever, and will be able to maintain his health on a cholesterol lowering regimen. As one can imagine, Mr. Schatz is thrilled with External CounterPulsation, as is his family.

William Pischke

William Pischke will be 72 years old this year—twenty years older than he ever dreamed he would be. Mr. Pischke assumed he would follow the same short path his parents and grandparents did, exhibiting early signs of heart disease and dying before age 50 of a heart attack or stroke.

Indeed, he did follow their path for some time, experiencing angina and shortness of breath in his 30s and submitting without blinking to his first open heart surgery at age 41.

Following surgery, Mr. Pischke went on a very regimented

exercise and diet program and did fairly well for approximately 18 years. In 1988 at the age of 59, he began experiencing increasingly severe angina. Two years later he had his second coronary artery bypass surgery in 1990 at the age of 61. This time he did well for only 7 years, when the symptoms of angina, shortness of breath, and coronary heart disease returned. He had to give up his pastime of playing tennis because of the severity of the chest pains. He also had to give up his daily walking and exercise routine. Mr Pischke was a prisoner in his own home limited to sedentary activities. In fact, just walking one block would cause extreme fatigue and angina.

Re-evaluation by his doctor suggested the need for a third open heart surgery, to which Mr. Pischke reluctantly agreed. However, in the operating room, upon cutting Mr. Pischke's chest open the doctors found so much scar tissue that they were unable to complete any bypasses at all. Mr. Pischke was sent home and told to be extremely cautious and that he might die at any time. It seemed there was nothing else modern medicine had to offer to him. Mr. Pischke's doctor prescribed all kinds of heart medication in an attempt to prevent a heart attack and give Mr. Pischke whatever relief might be possible.

This is when the Pischke's found out about External CounterPulsation therapy from a friend. Both Mr. Pischke and his wife were extremely skeptical that something so simple, safe and drug free would have any effect at all on someone as critically ill as himself. But at this point Mr. Pischke was willing to try anything! The surgeons and traditional cardiologists had nothing else to offer. Mr. Pischke wanted to be able to celebrate his upcoming 72nd birthday and be able to enjoy his grandchildren.

Under the careful direction of a physician trained in External CounterPulsation, Mr. Pischke began a course of treatment with ECP. He underwent an hour of treatment every day, 5 days a week for several weeks. After treatment with ECP Mr. Pischke was able to walk five miles without any difficulty, play some limited doubles tennis with friends and for the first time in years go on extended bicycle rides.

Today he cannot remember the last time that he needed nitroglycerin. The only medications he takes at this time are to keep his triglycerides less than 100, cholesterol at less than 150 and his LDL at less than 90.

Although Mr. Pischke cannot play tennis or walk like he did 20 years ago, he is significantly better than he was 2 years ago. In fact, Mr. Pischke and his wife strongly believe that if it were not for the External CounterPulsation treatment he might not even be alive today. This month Mr. Pischke celebrates his 72nd birthday and is optimistic that he will have many more birthdays to celebrate.

Dale Hall

Nine stents later and on maximum drug therapy, 57-year-old Mr. Hall still suffered from daily angina and excessive fatigue. Moreover, the only way Mr. Hall could get through a day at work was to take an extended lunch during which he napped for one to two hours. Fortunately, he is self- employed and can take time off in the middle of the day without requesting permission from a superior.

The interesting thing about Mr. Hall is that follow-up angiograms showed his stents were all open. However a thallium scan showed major circulation defects in the heart muscle. So what was causing the fatigue and angina? Mr. Hall's cardiologist told him it was coming from the blockage of many small coronary vessels too narrow to be bypassed, stented or angioplastied. Aware that nothing else could be done, he referred Mr. Hall to me for ECP. After seven weeks of ECP, Mr. Hall states that he is feeling excellent, is free of angina, and no longer needs to take naps during the day. A repeat treadmill and thallium scan done after ECP is now completely normal.

Neil Medford

Mr. Medford's story begins as a tragedy of errors. In 1993 at age 69, Mr. Medford went to his doctor with angina. Diagnosed with coronary artery disease, he submitted to his first angioplasty. In the summer of the following year the angina returned and angioplasty was once again performed on the same coronary artery. Mr. Medford lived virtually symptom-free until June of 1999 when the pain recurred, this time more severe than in the past. Stents were now in fashion, so the cardiologist placed three of them into the coronary arteries. Less than five months later, all the stents were found to have closed off. Now he was told it was time for triple bypass surgery, which did relieve Mr. Medford's pain—briefly. Just six months later the angina had returned, this time so severe as to substantially limit his lifestyle. You see, Mr. Medford had a small farm he enjoyed working on, and just about anything he tried to do would cause chest pain. Being out in the cold would bring on angina; walking up the slightest incline would cause serious chest pain and fatigue; even walking on level ground into the wind would cause Mr. Medford to slow down in pain. This time his cardiologist told him nothing more could be done, that he should take it easy and take his pills. Mr. Medford went home seriously depressed, fearing that he would have to spend the rest of his days as an invalid, staying at home.

There was one option left, however, one that Mr. Medford had found out about quite accidentally. Although there were no physicians in his town that offered ECP Mr. Medford found a clinic that provided treatment about 75 miles away. Anxious to get started, he began treatments the following month. After completing seven weeks of ECP, Mr. Medford returned to his farm and wrote us a wonderful letter. He wrote that he is almost entirely free of angina even after engaging in rather strenuous activity at the farm. At no time does he have to cease activity, nor has he developed any shortness of breath. He went on to say that he is now able to walk a mile rather rapidly without any angina. His letter to us concludes by stating that the results of the ECP treatment have been marvelous and that the fears he had of a severely restricted lifestyle have been erased. Mr. Medford now is looking forward to more active participation in life's physical endeavors.

Tom Wilson

Mr. Wilson, accompanied by his wife, came to my office huffing and puffing, pulling an oxygen cart beside him. It was a struggle for the 76-year-old retired stockbroker just to cross the few feet from the handicap parking space into the building. Even with the oxygen flowing at maximum levels, he had to stop three times along the way to catch his breath. His cardiologist as well as two cardiac surgeons had just told him that he needed bypass surgery without delay. You see, Mr. Wilson had been diagnosed with severe congestive heart failure and had an ejection fraction of only 15-20 percent. As if this were not enough, he was also significantly overweight and diabetic. Although his physicians insisted that surgery was his only option, they also told Mr. Wilson that a 20 percent or higher chance existed that he would not survive the operation and that if he did survive, he would be at high risk for postoperative stroke and/or kidney failure.

Of course Mr. Wilson and his wife had asked if there were not anything else that could be done. What about ECP, they asked? They were told that ECP was not what he needed and that Mr. Wilson would be scheduled for surgery later in the week. Mr. Wilson asked my opinion. Was he a candidate for ECP, or should he go through with the surgery? I told him that he was indeed a good candidate for ECP, that the latest research was showing excellent results in patients diagnosed with CHF. I reminded him that if for some reason ECP did not help him, he could still submit to the surgery.

Mr. Wilson came faithfully to the office every day after that first meeting, pulling his oxygen cart along beside him, eager to receive his ECP treatments. Progress was slow but steady, and by the end of two treatment cycles (70 treatments), he was substantially better. With an improved ejection fraction, Mr. Wilson's lungs were now receiving higher volumes of blood to replenish with oxygen and return to his oxygen-starved heart. As a result, he no longer needed his oxygen tank to make the walk into the treatment room and at home was able to walk a slow mile with little difficulty. Such an excursion would have been impossible prior to his receiving ECP. Mr. Wilson and his wife now simply refer to the ECP unit as the "miracle machine."

David Johnson

Seventy-six-year-old Mr. Johnson came to me for a second opinion about treatment options for his angina after his daughter, a nurse, told him of ECP. He had recently seen his family physician, an internist, and his cardiologist, neither of whom had told him about ECP. You see, Mr. Johnson suffers with almost daily episodes of angina and easy fatigability. Once an avid sportsman, he misses the simple pleasure of fishing in the stream that runs behind his mountain cottage. A treadmill test done over one and a half years ago showed abnormalities suggesting that his heart was not getting enough oxygen. An independent thinker, Mr. Johnson did not let the doctors scare him into surgery or angioplasty even though that is what had been recommended. The thought of surgery was just too frightening. He told me he would rather live with the angina if there weren't a safer alternative.

An evaluation and review of Mr Johnson's records showed that he was an excellent candidate for ECP. Upon completion of 35 sessions of ECP Mr. Johnson noticed a significant increase in his energy and can now do most activities without angina. He can now do things he never dreamed that he would be able to do again such as work out in the yard, go to the mall and play with his grandchildren and of course go fishing in the mountains.

*Note: The above stories are from real people however, their names have been changed. Since everybody is different individual results obtained from ECP will vary.

Chapter 3

Vital Information About Your Heart

What are the symptoms of a heart attack?

Usually when someone has a heart attack they will notice one or more of the following symptoms. These symptoms are very similar to angina except that they do not go away in a few minutes:

- Uncomfortable pressure, fullness, squeezing or pain in the center of the chest lasting more than 30 minutes

- Tight band around the chest or the feeling of an elephant sitting on the chest that won't go away

- Pressure or numbness or tingling sensation can spread to the left arm and into the jaw and neck

- Chest discomfort along with light-headedness, sweating, nausea, fainting or shortness of breath may also occur

Other symptoms that are less commonly associated with a heart attack are as follows:

Stomach or abdominal pain, feelings of indigestion or heart burn, nausea or dizziness, shortness of breath or a smothering sensation with difficulty breathing, anxiety, weakness, fatigue, palpitations, cold sweat or paleness. Not all of these symptoms will occur in every heart attack. Sometimes they come and go.

What is a heart attack?

   A heart attack is also referred to as myocardial infarction, myocardial thrombosis or coronary artery thrombosis. A heart attack develops when the blood supply to the heart muscle is greatly reduced or stopped. This usually occurs when the right coronary artery, the left anterior descending or left circumflex coronary artery is somehow blocked. This blockage can be from the build up of plaque due to atherosclerosis or it can be the result of the sudden formation of a blood clot that shuts off the blood supply in a coronary artery. This is referred to as coronary artery thrombosis or acute coronary occlusion. Sudden and unpredictable rupture, cracking or fissuring of an atherosclerotic plaque in an artery with minimal blockage (less than 50% blockage) can also occur leading to the development of an immediate blood clot which prevents blood flow through the coronary artery. Sometimes the coronary artery will contract or go into spasm. When an artery narrows or goes into spasm the blood supply is severely reduced or cut off. This can reverse itself but if it doesn't, it may lead to a severe heart attack and even death.

   The result of blockage or reduction of blood supply to the heart muscle leads to myocardial infarction, which is simply a medical term for damage or death of an area in the heart muscle. If the blood supply is only cut off temporarily, the heart muscle can recover. However if the blood supply is cut off for an extended period of time the heart will suffer permanent injury and some muscle cells will die. If this happens, scar tissue will take the place of the dead heart muscle cells which will result in the heart not being able to function or pump as effectively as it did prior to the damage.

What does angina or angina pectoris feel like?

   Angina pectoris, (literally pain in chest) referred to as simply angina, is the medical term used to describe chest pain due to spasms or blockages occurring in the coronary arteries. Angina refers to a condition in which the heart muscle does not receive enough blood and oxygen resulting in chest discomfort. Angina happens anytime there is not enough blood flow supplying oxygen to the heart muscle. It may happen during physical exercise, during or after eating especially large meals, when experiencing strong emotions, or during extreme temperatures, for instance when it's very hot or very cold outside. In people with severe blockages angina may occur during sitting or when lying down.

Angina symptoms usually last only 1 to 5 minutes and can include some or all of the following:

- Vague chest discomfort

- Chest burning, pressure, squeezing, crushing, heaviness, smothering or indigestion, often described as a tight band around the chest or like someone is sitting on the chest

- Discomfort can radiate to the jaw, neck, arm, or shoulders, presented as a numbness or tingling sensation.

Women will often complain of somewhat different symptoms than men. When women are having angina they are more likely to complain of:

- Abdominal or digestive pain

- Shortness of breath

- Nausea and vomiting

- Fatigue.

Coronary artery spasm, also known as Prinzmetal's angina, occurs almost only at rest and is due to a sudden spasm of the coronary artery. The spasm usually occurs close to an obstructed or partially blocked blood vessel.

Stenosis and restenosis of coronary arteries.

It is important to understand stenosis and restenosis of coronary arteries since this is a very common occurrence after angioplasty, stent placement and even coronary artery bypass surgery. Stenosis is simply a medical term that means constriction or narrowing of a blood vessel. A coronary artery that has fat and cholesterol deposits built up in it is said to be constricted or narrowed; this is also referred to as stenosis. One procedure for widening or opening the coronary artery is percutaneous transluminal coronary angioplasty (PTCA) or angioplasty for short. About one third or more of patients that undergo PTCA have restenosis of the widened segment of the blood vessel within six months of the procedure. Restenosis simply means that the previously opened blood vessel has now closed down or narrowed again. Restenosis not only occurs after angioplasty and stents but it can also occur after coronary artery bypass graft (CABG).

Coronary artery bypass graft is a type of heart surgery where new blood vessels are sewn in to bypass blood around clogged arteries and improve the supply of blood and oxygen to the heart. Doctors often use the saphenous vein from the leg or the mammary artery from the chest in order to perform these bypass surgeries. It should be noted that the blood vessels used to bypass blocked areas might also become blocked.

How is angina classified?

In order to be able to compare the degree of angina from one patient to another researchers developed a standard way of describing angina. The Canadian Heart Classification is the most often used guide to describe a person's limitation from angina pectoris.

CANADIAN HEART CLASSIFICATION of ANGINA

CLASS I. Ordinary physical activity, such as walking and climbing stairs, does not cause angina. Angina occurs with strenuous, rapid or prolonged exertion during work or recreational activity.

CLASS II. Slight limitations of ordinary activity by angina. Angina occurs when walking or climbing stairs rapidly, walking uphill, walking or climbing stairs after meals, in the cold, against the wind, under emotional stress, for the first few hours after awakening. Angina pectoris may also occur when walking more than 2 blocks on level ground at sea level and climbing more than one flight or level of house stairs at your normal pace and in a comfortable environment.

CLASS III. Marked limitation of normal physical activity. Angina pectoris occurs when walking one to two blocks on level ground and climbing one flight of stairs under normal conditions and at normal pace (not too cold, hot or windy, at sea level).

CLASS IV. Inability to carry on any physical activity without anginal discomfort. Angina may be present at rest.

Summarized it is as follows:

Class	Activity that makes you have Angina	Limits of Activity
I	Prolonged excessive exercise.	No limitation of normal activity.
II	Walking more than 2 blocks.	Slight limitation of normal activity.
III	Walking less than 2 blocks.	Normal activity is significantly limited.
IV	Minimal activity or while resting.	Severe limitation of normal activity.

What is atherosclerosis?
"Athero-" is Greek for paste and "-sclerosis" simply refers to hardness. Atherosclerosis refers to the deposits of fat, cholesterol, calcium and clotting factors that buildup in the inner lining of arteries. These substances also act as irritants to the lining of the blood vessels. This insult to the artery then leads to excessive growth of muscle cells in the blood vessel lining, which further reduces blood flow in the artery. Physicians often refer to this accumulation as plaque. If this atherosclerotic plaque becomes large enough it can reduce blood flow and cause a heart attack or stroke.

Atherosclerosis is a slow process that often starts in childhood. There are many factors that are thought to contribute to damage of the blood vessel lining.
- High levels of LDL cholesterol
- High levels of triglycerides
- Insulin resistance
- High blood pressure
- Smoking
- Elevated homocysteine
- Elevated Lp(a)

These factors are discussed in greater detail later in the book.

Tests for heart disease.
We have all seen TV shows and movies where doctors or paramedics place paddles on a person's chest and tell everyone nearby to "stand clear." We have seen patients start breathing again after these paddles have been applied and the heart beats again. However, what many may not realize is that the reason these charged paddles work is because the heart is an electrically controlled muscle, as a jolt of lightning may kill a person, a controlled jolt of electricity may restore a person back to life, by "jump starting" the heart.

Electrocardiogram

When we want to find out how the heart is functioning as an electrical unit, we use a machine that measures and records the electrical impulses in different areas of the heart. Just as a wall thermostat measures the temperature of the air in your house and provides a numeric reading, a doctor measures the electrical impulses of the heart with a machine and the reading it provides is called an electrocardiogram.

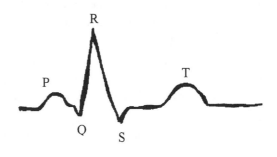

In your house, you may have thermometers in more than one place. The temperature in your kitchen is most likely warmer than other rooms because of the heat given off by the oven and other appliances. When a doctor measures the electrical impulses of the heart, he takes these measurements in different areas too. To do this, he uses long wires called "leads." Attached to the ends of these wires are little pads that are placed on certain areas of the patient's chest. Sometimes the doctor may use three leads; sometimes twelve. The readings obtained by the pads are sent to a machine that prints the findings on a piece of graph paper.

An electrocardiogram is often abbreviated ECG (sometimes also abbreviated EKG after the German elektrokardiogramm). The lines that are printed on an ECG look similar to the lines from a lie detector machine. Just like the police officer can tell by the changes in the lines whether someone is lying or not, the doctor can tell by the changes in the ECG lines whether the heart is healthy or whether it has suffered a previous heart attack. The electrical rhythm of your heart can also be determined from an ECG.

The ECG patterns have different names. One pattern has a definite shape and is called an "ST segment depression". An ST segment depression is seen when an area of the heart is lacking oxygen. The good news is that ST segment depressions are reversible and are no longer seen on follow-up ECG when the heart has received additional oxygen.

Another pattern often observed on an ECG is called a "Q" wave. This pattern indicates that the heart has been damaged and is seen when the patient has had a previous heart attack. Often times, the patient is totally unaware that they have even had the heart attack but the ECG results provide this important information to the doctor.

Echocardiogram

Just as the word "echo" implies this test uses sound waves to obtain information about the heart. A technician applies a small amount of gel to the patient's chest and moves a handle shaped device in the gel over the chest. The sound waves record an actual picture of the heart that is viewed on a TV-like monitor. This test can provide your doctor with a lot of valuable information without the use of x-rays, needles or dyes.

The echocardiogram provides information that is unobtainable from an ECG. An ECG provides an electrical picture of the heart while the echocardiogram provides a mechanical assessment of how the heart muscle and valves are functioning. The pictures of the heart that are shown with this test includes both the outside and inside of the heart. The doctor is able to see the size and shape of the heart as well as the inside chambers and individual valves in the heart. The doctor can evaluate the movement of the heart muscle, the movement of the valves, and the size of the heart chambers.

Ejection fraction

Another very important piece of information the doctor is able to obtain from an echocardiogram is called the ejection fraction. This is the amount or percentage of blood that is ejected or pumped out of the heart with each beat. A well functioning heart should pump out at least 50% of the blood with each beat. So, if a heart has 100ml of blood in it and 50ml was pumped out with one beat, the heart would have an ejection fraction of 50%. An ejection fraction of 50% or higher is considered a normal percent and would indicate that there is probably no need for treatment. However, if the ejection fraction is less than 50%, the heart is most likely not getting enough oxygen and not enough blood from the coronary arteries. In this situation, a doctor would most likely suggest the need for treatment, usually consisting of bypass surgery or angioplasty. However, External CounterPulsation (ECP) may be a better option!

Thallium or Cardiolite®(Du Pont Pharmaceuticals) (technetium-Tc99m sestamibi) Scans

This test is performed to measure blood flow to the heart muscle and is most often done in combination with an exercise treadmill stress test. The benefit of combining these two tests is that blood flow to the heart can be monitored and evaluated prior to exercise, immediately following exercise, and then a few hours later. A small amount of radioactive tracer material called thallium or technetium-99m is injected into the bloodstream either prior to or while the patient is walking on the treadmill. As the blood circulates through the body the tracer is circulated with it. The cells of the heart muscle have a strong affinity toward the tracer and absorb it readily, more so than any other cells in the body. The patient then lies down on a table under a special camera that is able to capture images of the tracer in the heart. By looking at these pictures the doctor can see which parts of the heart are getting adequate blood supply and which parts are not. If a portion of the heart is getting too little blood, that area will reveal a decreased amount of the tracer and show up as a dark area on the film. Heart muscle that is getting sufficient blood will show up as light areas on the film.

If this procedure is done prior to exercise then the patient starts walking on the treadmill and repeats the picture taking process immediately following exercise. The doctor can compare the before and after exercise tracer scans. Sometimes the scan shows that the heart is getting enough blood during rest, but not enough during exercise. This may be due to blockages or spasms in the coronary arteries. In other patients there will be low amounts of tracer in the heart prior to and after exercise, which would indicate that the heart has poor circulation all the time. If there is no tracer at all seen in a portion of the heart muscle it is because the heart has scar tissue from a previous heart attack and the muscle cells in this particular part of the heart have died. Comparison scans done before and after a course of ECP often show a dramatic improvement in circulation.

Ultrafast CT Electron Beam Tomography

Ultrafast computerized tomography or ultrafast CT is a quick, painless test that can be very useful as a screening tool in the diagnosis of coronary artery disease. Ultrafast CT uses x-rays to reveal the amount of calcium in the blood vessels around the heart. The greater the amount of calcium seen the more likely that there is significant coronary artery disease. Although a high concentration of calcium in these vessels does suggest the strong possibility of blockage, it does not pinpoint nor confirm the location or certainty of a blockage. Additional testing is necessary to determine if circulation to the heart is impaired. Ultrafast CT can be a valuable tool in evaluating patients at risk for heart disease. Dr. Robert H. Eckel, Professor of Medicine, University of Colorado School of Medicine states, "…the diagnosis of coronary disease can be made pretty quickly with this test…it has changed my practice."

If the calcium score is elevated then aggressive risk factor modification is usually necessary.

For more information, you may contact Colorado Heart Imaging at 800-800-3943 or 303-433-8800.

References:
Fallavollita JA, Brody AS, Bunnell IL, et al. Fast computed tomography detection of coronary calcification in the diagnosis of coronary artery disease. Comparison with angiography in patients<50 years old. Circulation 1994 Jan;89(1):285-90.

Chapter 4

What Angiograms
Can't Tell You

A *cardiac* angiogram (also known as a cardiac catheterization) is ordered to provide your doctor with 4 pieces of information:

1. Blood pressure in the heart
2. Pumping ability of the heart muscle, also known as the ejection fraction of the heart
3. Amount of oxygen in the blood
4. How blood is flowing through the heart itself and how the valves function.

This procedure is done in the hospital outpatient center and is performed by a physician. A local anesthetic is given and a tiny, flexible tube called a catheter, is placed through the skin and into an artery, usually in the groin. During this 30 minute procedure, a TV like monitor and motion x-rays are used to assist the doctor in guiding the tube towards the heart and finally to the coronary arteries.

If the doctor wishes to see areas of blockage or poor circulation, dye is injected into the catheter and up to the coronary arteries. When this dye is used, the procedure is called a *coronary* angiography or *coronary* arteriography. During this procedure the doctor can estimate blockages in the coronary arteries.

The catheter may have a balloon on the tip of it which the doctor can inflate in a blood vessel that has a small blockage. The ballooning expands the artery and results in increased blood flow. This balloon procedure is called percutaneous transluminal coronary angioplasty or PTCA for short. Percutaneous means "through the skin," transluminal coronary means "into the opening of the coronary artery," and angioplasty means "widening of the blood vessel." In recent years doctors have added the placement of stents to the coronary angioplasty treatment.

Where are you in the statistics?

In 1992, several doctors from Harvard University Medical School conducted a study, and the results were published in the *Journal of the American Medical Association.* One hundred-sixty-eight patients had been recently examined by other doctors and were diagnosed as requiring cardiac angiography. These 168 patients were then referred to the teaching hospital in Boston, Massachusetts for a second opinion.

Upon evaluation of these 168 patients by the Harvard doctors, 134 or 80% were determined not to require angiography and 28 or 17% had the angiography postponed until further studies could be done. Only 6 out of the original patients or 4% were actually determined to require the procedure.

The Harvard physicians concluded that the majority of patients presenting with coronary heart disease whose conditions were medically stable, could safely postpone coronary angiography. Furthermore, the doctors also stated that it would be reasonable to estimate that 50% of all coronary angiographies done in this country are unnecessary at the present time and could at the very least be postponed.

Can angiograms tell which blood vessels will cause a heart attack?

Bowman Gray School of Medicine published a study in 1988 in the journal of the American Heart Association, *Circulation,* which looked at how well (or how poorly) angiograms predicted the site of future myocardial infarctions or "heart attacks." We need to remember that the supposed purpose of an angiogram is to determine which coronary arteries are blocked, to what degree and what course of action is required to correct these problems.

The findings of the study indicated that through angiograms doctors were able to predict which coronary artery blockages would lead to a heart attack only 34% of the time. Sixty-six percent of the time the blood vessel that caused a heart attack was less than 50% blocked at the time of angiography. (It is interesting to note that it is possible to run a marathon with all three major coronary vessels blocked by 50%.)

They found that 97% of the time the blood vessels responsible for heart attacks were less than 70% blocked. Only 34% of the time did a heart attack occur as a result of a blood vessel that was found to be the most blocked during an angiogram. The doctors concluded that angiograms are inadequate in predicting the time or location of a blockage that will result in a heart attack. Furthermore, the authors state that usually a heart attack results from a blockage that was not considered at the time to be dangerous. Put very simply this means that while blood vessels that are 80 to 90% blocked cause angina, it is the blood vessels that are less than 70% blocked that are the ones most likely to cause a heart attack! In other words, a heart attack is more likely to be caused by a non critical or small lesion than a large so called critical lesion!

The reason that these small lesions or plaque are so dangerous is due to the fact that they may rupture. When a 40% blockage ruptures a blood clot forms over the rupture and what was once an inconsequential blockage grows quickly, in a matter of minutes, from 40% to 100%. This rapid occlusion causes severe angina and if not immediately treated may cause a heart attack. Angioplasty and stents do not prevent unstable plaque from rupturing. This may partly explain the high failure rate of these procedures.

Another study was published in 1994 in the *Annals of Internal Medicine*. This study set out to answer the question: What are the limitations of angiography in analyzing coronary atherosclerosis? The researchers determined the following:

1. Coronary angiography does not measure atherosclerosis.

2. Angiography cannot tell you what is in the build up that causes blockages. This is important because the chemistry of certain plaques makes them more unstable and subsequently more likely to rupture.

3. Angiography does not show the mechanical properties of the blockage. A blockage that puts a lot of stress-strain on the arterial wall is more likely to rupture than one that does not.

4. Angiography does not help in any way to predict the likelihood that a coronary artery plaque or blockage will rupture, causing a blood clot and subsequent heart attack.

5. The so-called "normal" reference blood vessels which doctors use to compare to the blocked or narrowed artery may in fact not be normal.

6. The images obtained from an angiography are two dimensional and in reality the coronary arteries are three-dimensional. Blood vessels twist and turn and overlap making the doctor's interpretation quite difficult. (A comparison can be made to sitting in front of a bowl of spaghetti. Looking down into the bowl, it is very difficult to determine where one piece of spaghetti starts, where it goes and where it ends.)

7. There is no standardization of the techniques that doctors use to study angioplasty and to estimate the percentage of blockage.

8. The severity or occurrence of angina *cannot* be predicted by a blockage seen on an angiogram.

9. It is very difficult to determine whether existing atherosclerosis is getting better or worse.

X-rays and inconsistent readings.

The *New England Journal of Medicine* published an interesting article in 1984, which documented x-ray readings given by doctors. The intent of the study was to see if different doctors would agree on the size of the blockages and if they could accurately predict the magnitude of coronary artery stenosis by viewing only the x-rays taken during the procedures.

Coronary angiograms belonging to several different patients were shown to a group of doctors. The patient's names were covered so the doctors did not know whose x-rays or "films" they were reviewing. The same films were shown to the same doctors on different occasions. The same films were also shown to a different group of doctors and the results were compared.

The study revealed that 95% of the time there were inaccuracies in estimating the extent of coronary blockage even when the same doctor read the same film but on a different day. The authors concluded that the viewing of angiograms by doctors was ineffective in evaluating or estimating coronary blockages.

"But my doctor told me..."

"My doctor told me I need an angiogram to diagnose coronary artery disease."

If you have angina pectoris or have had a heart attack, it is already known that you have coronary heart disease. Further testing is usually unnecessary.

"My doctor told me that before he gives me any medication, he needs to know what my coronary arteries look like."

It is not necessary to know what the blood vessels look like in order to prescribe medication. A thorough medical history and perhaps an exercise test yield sufficient information to prescribe appropriate medication, if indicated. If you are presently taking medication or have done External CounterPulsation and have relief of your angina then there is no need for further testing.

"My doctor told me that until he sees what my blood vessels look like, he cannot give me a prognosis."

Research has clearly shown that a prognosis is determined by the efficiency of the pumping ability of the left ventricle. If the left ventricle pumps with a 50% or greater efficiency ("ejection fraction"), the prognosis is good. The ejection fraction is a much more valuable piece of information than how many blood vessels are diseased. An ejection fraction can be easily and safely obtained from an echocardiogram.

"My doctor told me that a coronary angiogram will tell him if I have a seriously blocked vessel that could cause me to have a heart attack."

Research has shown that the severely blocked blood vessels are *not* the ones most likely to cause a heart attack.

When does an angiogram need to be done?
- When there is a substantial drop in blood pressure or a severe ECG change during a treadmill test

- When angina at rest cannot be controlled with medications

- When angina is accompanied by fluid in the lungs

- When a patient is unable to tolerate medications

- When angina is accompanied by a dangerous cardiac rhythm.

References:

Graboys TB, Biegelsen B, Lampert S, et al. Results of a second-opinion trial among patients recommended for coronary angiography. JAMA 1992 Nov 11;268(18):2537-40.

Little WC, Constantinescu M, Applegate RJ, et al. Can coronary angiography predict the site of a subsequent myocardial infarction in patients with mild-to-moderate coronary artery disease? Circulation 1988 Nov;78 (5 Pt 1):1157-1166.

White CW, Wright CB , Doty DB, et al. Does visual interpretation of the coronary arteriogram predict the physiologic importance of a coronary stenosis? N Engl J Med 1984 Mar 29;310(13):819-824.

Hong MK, Mintz GS, Popma JJ, et al. Limitations of angiography for analyzing coronary atherosclerosis progression or regression. Ann Intern Med 1994 Sep 1;121(5):348-354.

Topol EJ, Nissen SE. Our preoccupation with coronary luminology. The dissociation between clinical and angiographic findings in ischemic heart disease. Circulation 1995 Oct 15;92(8):2333-2342.

Chapter 5

Angioplasty, Doctors Weaned on the Quick Fix

Why Angioplasty is Not the Answer

Angioplasty is known by many names including balloon angioplasty, coronary angioplasty, coronary artery angioplasty, angioplasty of the heart, PTCA or Percutaneous Transluminal Coronary Angioplasty. However, after reading this book you will realize that ECP is changing the interpretation of PTCA to: Put That Catheter Away and give me ECP, External Counter Pulsation instead!

Regardless of which name is used the procedure remains the same. Angioplasty is a catheterization laboratory procedure performed by a cardiologist in an effort to widen a narrowed coronary artery. A catheter with a specialized inflatable balloon tip is passed into the "stenosed" or narrowed part of the artery. The doctor then gently blows up the balloon tip and attempts to widen the narrow area. Although this procedure is considered easier and less traumatic than bypass surgery, there remains the potential for severe complications. Arteries may rupture during the balloon inflation, develop an aneurysm or may simply tear during the catheter procedure. When this occurs the only option is to perform an emergency coronary artery bypass.

It is interesting to note that the American College of Cardiology defines a successful angioplasty as follows:

If a blood vessel is made 20% bigger with angioplasty and is less than 50% blocked after the angioplasty then it is considered a successful procedure! In other words, if you had a blood vessel that was 79 % blocked and your doctor was able to decrease the blockage by 30% so that now the blood vessel was only 49% blocked, this would be considered a success even though your blood vessel is still 49% blocked. Without further treatment the chances are good that the blockage will re-occur.

Medications or surgery, pick one.

One of the premier medical institutions in America is the Mayo Clinic. In 1997 *The Mayo Clinic Proceedings* published a comparison article discussing the long-term outcomes of coronary angioplasty for unstable angina and angina pain that occurred while at rest between men and women. The women had a 13% failure rate when undergoing angioplasty. The in-hospital death rate was 25% higher for women undergoing angioplasty than it was for men. As for emergency bypass surgery, which was needed as a result of an angioplasty that didn't go well, 3% of the women and 3.5% of the men ended up having emergency coronary bypass surgery as a result of a failed angioplasty. The six-year death rate was 19% for women and 15% for men. After six years 19% of the women and 22% of the men needed coronary artery bypass surgery. Within six years 52% of the women and 44% of the men had reoccurrence of severe angina.

Baylor Medical College in Houston Texas conducted a study comparing patients that had angioplasty with other patients that had intensive medication therapy. In November of 1998, the American Heart Association published the findings in their official journal, *Circulation.*

The patients studied were stable survivors of heart attacks. Some of the patients were given angioplasty and the others were given aggressive therapy with medication. The authors discovered that either intensive medical therapy (prescription drugs) or angioplasties were equally effective in relieving angina symptoms in patients who had recovered from a previous heart attack.

A more recent study published in the July 8, 1999 issue of the *New England Journal of Medicine* reported on 341 patients that were treated either with angioplasties or with atorvastatin (Lipitor,™ Parke Davis). Atorvastatin is a powerful medicine that is used by physicians to lower cholesterol. One half of the patients that had coronary artery disease were treated with angioplasties and the other half of the patients were treated with enough atorvastatin to bring the LDL cholesterol down to below 75 milligrams for a continuous period of 18 months. At the end of the study the researchers found that those patients taking atorvastatin had 36% fewer heart symptoms and needed less surgery for angina than patients who had undergone angioplasty. The researchers concluded that aggressive reduction of LDL cholesterol with medication is at least as *effective* as angioplasty for coronary artery disease patients. Dr. Pitt, one of the authors, went on to state that none of the patients in the atorvastatin group suffered by not undergoing angioplasty and if needed they could still have angioplasty performed later.

Is this success?

In the *American Journal of Cardiology* 1992 the Mid-American Heart Institute from Kansas City, Missouri published a study where they looked at what happened to patients two years after they had had angioplasty. What they found was both interesting and disappointing. Immediately after the angioplasty procedure was completed it appeared to be 95% successful. So no need to worry? Wrong! The doctors found that within two years of angioplasty 49% of patients had to have a repeat cardiac catheterization. Within two years of angioplasty 30% of the patients had to have a repeat angioplasty, 23% of the patients went on to have coronary artery bypass graft, also known as CABG and 10% of the patients died. In other words, within two years, 53% of the patients had to have additional surgery.

Is the grass greener down under?

In 1994, in the same journal, researchers from Queensland,

Australia didn't have any better results to report. In this study doctors found that five years after angioplasty 80% of patients still had angina and 33% of patients needed repeat surgery. During angioplasty three percent of the patients had complications that required emergency bypass surgery. By the end of the five year study three percent of the angioplasty patients died.

Are the Europeans more successful?

Let's take a look at a study published in the *Journal of the American College of Cardiology* completed at Erasmus University in Rotterdam, the Netherlands. In this study researchers looked at 856 patients that had percutaneous transluminal coronary angioplasty (PTCA) 10 years later. The results are not encouraging. After ten years 47% of the patients had a return of the same symptoms for which they originally had surgery, 60% still needed to take medications for their angina and another 43% had either a heart attack, bypass surgery, repeat angioplasty or died in the 10 years following their first angioplasty. The official summary that the doctors arrived at is perplexing. The doctors reviewing this study concluded that the long-term outcome of angioplasty is good but that the majority of patients will experience further cardiac problems within ten years. So which is it? Maybe what they meant is that the outcome is good for the practicing cardiologist because they keep you coming back?

Let's review another study done in Europe. This one was published in 1992 and was done in the Department of Cardiology in Holland. The doctors in this study looked at long term results of angioplasty in patients that were 75 years of age and older. After successful angioplasty, they found that 75% of the patients had a return of their same heart symptoms within seven years. It is evident that the Europeans don't have any better success with angioplasty than we do.

How does coronary artery bypass graft or CABG compare to angioplasty?

In 1994 the *New England Journal of Medicine* published a study that was completed in Hamburg, Germany. Let's see if the Germans have any better success than the Americans or Australians in treating coronary artery disease. In this study 177 patients were treated with CABG and 182 patients were treated with PTCA also known as angioplasty. The patients were only studied for one year and the results were as follows: 2.3% of the angioplasty patients had a heart attack during angioplasty and 8% of the CABG patients had a heart attack during bypass surgery. While in the hospital 2.5% of the CABG patients died compared to 1.1% of the angioplasty patients. Repeat CABG treatment within the first year was necessary for 6% of the CABG patients while 44% of the angioplasty patients had to go back in the first year for repeat angioplasty. After one year 78% of the CABG patients continued to need medications for angina while 88% of the angioplasty patients needed medication for angina.

Take your pick: medication, angioplasty or bypass.

The inefficiency and ineffectiveness of angioplasty is well documented. But how do other treatment options compare to the highly overrated procedure of angioplasty? The *Journal of the American College of Cardiology* published an article in December of 1995, which answered this question.

The object of the study was to determine the effectiveness of three different procedures for the treatment of severe stenosis (narrowing) of the left anterior descending (LAD) artery in patients with angina. (Please refer to diagram in Chapter 9.) Patients at the Heart Institute of the University of Sao Paulo, Brazil were monitored for three years during and after their treatment for coronary artery disease. Some of the patients had received angioplasty; others had undergone bypass surgery; and others were treated only with medication.

At the end of the three-year study the researchers discovered that there was no difference found in the current symptoms or the recovery of the three different groups. Statistically, each group had the same amount of heart attacks, deaths, symptoms or improvements. The authors stated that this information should be taken into consideration when physicians are discussing therapeutic choices with their patients. Now with the addition of ECP you have four treatment choices for angina that your physician can discuss with you.

What treatment is best at getting you back to work?

Now back to the United States for the following study. This study was published in the *Annals of Internal Medicine* and the question was which patients will get back to work quicker? Will a patient who has had angioplasty, coronary bypass surgery or medical therapy be more likely to be back at work and employed one year later? This was a large study of 1252 patients who were all younger than 65 years of age. The outcome that these researchers from the Duke University Medical Center compared was how many patients were employed after one year. The investigation found that after one year 80% of the bypass patients were back to work, 84% of the angioplasty patients were back to work and 79% of the patients that underwent medical treatment only were back to work. The official conclusion was that neither surgery nor angioplasty improved the patients' ability to be back at work after one year any better than did medical therapy.

Who was able to get back to work sooner? Well, the patients that received only medicine were back to work within 14 days. Those patients that received angioplasty were able to return to work after 18 days and those patients who had coronary artery bypass surgery were generally able to return back to work within approximately 54 days. Keep in mind that External CounterPulsation can be done while you continue working and that no lengthy recovery or rehabilitation program is necessary. While the other treatments require more medications, treatment with ECP usually means you will be able to take fewer drugs!

Which arteries will become blocked faster?

The next study is fascinating because it looks at the natural history of coronary atherosclerosis using quantitative angiography in men. This was called the Harvard atherosclerosis reversibility project study group and was completed at Brigham and Woman's Hospital at Boston University in Boston Massachusetts. The researchers discovered that while doctors bypass or perform angioplasty on the most severely blocked arteries, it is the minimally blocked arteries that clog up more rapidly. This means that while everyone is worried about fixing that 95% blockage with angioplasty or a stent, it is the arteries that are only mildly diseased that are clogging at a much faster rate and statistically will be the ones most likely to cause you heart problems in the future.

The National Medicare Experience after angioplasty.

Any Medicare patient about to undergo non-emergency angioplasty should be aware of the following research completed by Dr. Eric Peterson and his associates at Duke University Medical Center. Unfortunately elderly patients are rarely quoted accurate figures. Please remember that this study looks only at the death rate after successful angioplasty. If strokes, kidney failure, infections and depression are also taken into account the rate of morbidity and mortality could easily exceed 50%. Don't be seduced by technology. The treatment you choose could be more hazardous to you than the heart disease. If medications, diet and ECP fail then angioplasty can always be attempted later.

The National Medicare Experience Death After Angioplasty in 225,915 Patients		
Ages	30 Day % death rate	1 Year % death rate
65-69	2.1	5.2
70-74	3.0	7.3
75-79	4.6	10.9
Greater than 80	7.8	17.3

Diabetics have poor outcome with angioplasty.
In the August 1999 issue of the *Journal of the American College of Cardiology*, Dr. Eric Van Belle reports on 485 diabetic patients that underwent angioplasty. The procedure was successful in 94% of the patients. However, the researchers were startled by the fact that after only six months 75% of the lesions were 50% or more blocked!

Angioplasty patients often need more bypass surgery!
The *British Journal of Medicine* recently released a comprehensive analysis of randomized controlled angioplasty trials published between 1979 and 1998. The analysis, performed by Swiss Dr. H.C. Bucher and colleagues, compared 953 patients who had undergone angioplasty with 951 patients who had received only medical treatment. The conclusions were startling. Angioplasty had reduced angina but at an exorbitant price. Patients who had undergone angioplasty were 29% more likely to need repeat angioplasty, 32% more apt to die, 42% more liable to have a heart attack and 59% more prone to need bypass surgery. The researchers themselves were at a loss to explain how a procedure thought to be helping patients is actually making them worse. In conclusion, Dr. Bucher recommended

that medical treatment be preferred over angioplasty for patients with stable coronary artery disease and that angioplasty be reserved for non-acute patients only after all else has failed. Why not try ECP first?

Why is it that angioplasty has such a poor success rate?

There are many recognized weaknesses of angioplasty. For example, during angioplasty your doctor cannot cross blockages. If there are two severe blockages in the same blood vessel, the doctor will not be able to cross through one blockage to get to the other blockage.

The doctor is unable to dilate blood vessels that have a lot of elasticity. Blood vessels that are very rubbery cannot be successfully dilated because they simply will not hold their shape. It is also common for an artery to be narrowed in more than one place, or for an artery to have a lengthy area of narrowing. When this occurs, it is impossible for the doctor to dilate (enlarge) more than one specific spot in the artery.

While dilating the blood vessel the cardiologist needs to be very careful not to over expand the artery so much that it will rupture or tear. If that should happen you will end up in the surgery suite undergoing an emergency coronary artery bypass graft. Bigger is not always better. Occasionally angioplasty causes aneurysms in the coronary artery.

Angioplasty is unable to prevent re-clogging or re-stenosis of the blood vessels that have been opened up. It is a quick and in many cases a temporary fix for only one or two blockages. Remember, it is impossible to tell just by looking at a blockage if it is a critical blockage or not.

Still want to do angioplasty?

If, after reading this you are still thinking about undergoing coronary angioplasty I would suggest you read further. In 1995 the University of Pennsylvania Hospital published a study in the *Journal of the American Medical Association* showing that there was a significant decrease in complications in hospitals that performed more than 600 angioplasties per year. Hospitals that did less than 200 angioplasties per year were compared to those that did more than 600 angioplasties per year. What became apparent was that hospitals doing more than 600 angioplasties a year had 46% fewer major complications than those performing less than 200 angioplasties per year.

Similar conclusions were again published in 1997 in the same *Journal of the American Medical Association.* This investigation was done at the State University of New York at Albany where researchers looked at coronary angioplasty and how the number of procedures done by the interventional cardiologist corresponded with how well the patient did. Cardiologists that did less than 75 angioplasties per year were compared to cardiologists that did more than 175 angioplasties per year. What these researchers found was doctors performing fewer than 75 angioplasties per year had patients that were 13% more likely to die during angioplasty. Furthermore they found that doctors who did 175 or more angioplasties per year were 38% less likely to have complications with their patients such as the need for emergency bypass surgery. The conclusion of the study was that the more experienced cardiologist had a lower hospital death rate and decreased need for emergency coronary artery bypass graft surgery.

The American College of Cardiology's current guidelines recommends that each cardiologist should perform at least 75 angioplasties per year in order to remain proficient. Unfortunately it is estimated that the average cardiologist today does fewer than 50 angioplasties per year.

In conclusion, there appears to be only two real advantages to angioplasty.

1. It can give immediate, life saving relief of angina during a heart attack.

2. It improves the angiographic *picture* of the coronary artery. Angioplasty *does not* prevent heart attacks and *does not* decrease the chances of dying from heart disease!

For chronic angina it is obvious that ECP has many advantages. Along with lipid lowering therapy ECP should be the treatment of choice for most patients.

PTCA: Put that catheter away

References:
Dakik HA , Kleiman NS, Farmer JA , et al. Intensive medical therapy versus coronary angioplasty for suppression of myocardial ischemia in survivors of acute myocardial infarction: a prospective, randomized pilot study. Circulation 1998 Nov 10;98(19):2017-2023.

Pitt B, Waters D, Brown WV, et al. Aggressive Lipid-Lowering Therapy Compared with Angioplasty in Stable Coronary Artery Disease. New Eng J Med—July 8, 1999 341(2):70-76.

Vacek JL, Rosamond TL, Stites HW, et al. Comparison of percutaneous transluminal coronary angioplasty versus coronary artery bypass grafting for multivessel coronary artery disease. Am J Cardiol 1992 Mar 1;69(6):592-597.

Cameron J, Mahanonda N, Aroney C, et al. Outcome five years after percutaneous transluminal coronary angioplasty or coronary artery bypass grafting for significant narrowing limited to the left anterior descending coronary artery. Am J Cardiol 1994 Sep 15;74(6):544-549.

Hamm CW, Reimers J, Ischinger T, et al. A randomized study of coronary angioplasty compared with bypass surgery in patients with symptomatic multivessel coronary disease. German Angioplasty Bypass Surgery Investigation. N Engl J Med 1994 Oct 20;331(16):1037-1043.

Hueb WA, Bellotti G, de Oliveira SA, et al. The Medicine, Angioplasty or Surgery Study (MASS): a prospective, randomized trial of medical therapy, balloon angioplasty or bypass surgery for single proximal left anterior descending artery stenoses. J Am Coll Cardiol 1995 Dec;26(7):1600-1605.

Mark DB, Lam LC, Lee KL, et al. Effects of coronary angioplasty, coronary bypass surgery, and medical therapy on employment in patients with coronary artery disease. A prospective comparison study. Ann Intern Med 1994 Jan 15;120(2):111-117.

Keelan ET, Nunez BD, Grill DE, et al. Comparison of immediate and long-term outcome of coronary angioplasty performed for unstable angina and rest pain in men and women. Mayo

Clin Proc 1997 Jan;72(1):5-12.

Ruygrok PN, de Jaegere PT, van Domburg RT, et al. Clinical outcome 10 years after attempted percutaneous transluminalcoronary angioplasty in 856 patients. J Am Coll Cardiol 1996 Jun;27(7):1669-1677.

Berg JM, Bal ET, Gin TJ, et al. Initial and long-term results of percutaneous transluminal coronary angioplasty in patients 75 years of age and older. Cathet Cardiovasc Diagn 1992 Jul;26(3):165-170.

Stone PH, Gibson CM, Pasternak RC, et al. Natural history of coronary atherosclerosis using quantitative angiography in men, and implications for clinical trials of coronary regression. The Harvard Atherosclerosis Reversibility Project Study Group. Am J Cardiol 1993 Apr 1;71(10):766-772.

Kimmel SE , Berlin JA , Laskey WK. The relationship between coronary angioplasty procedure volume and major complications. JAMA 1995 Oct 11;274(14):1137-1142.

Hannan EL, Racz M, Ryan TJ, et al. Coronary angioplasty volume-outcome relationships for hospitals and cardiologists. JAMA 1997 Mar 19;277(11):892-898.

Van Belle E. et al. Restenosis after angioplasty in diabetics. J Am Coll Cardiol 1999;34:476-485.

Bucher HC, et al. Percutaneous transluminal coronary angioplasty versus medical treatment for the non-acute coronary heart disease: meta-analysis of randomized controlled trials. BMJ 2000;321:73-7

Peterson ED, Jollis JG, Bebchuk JD, et al. Changes in mortality after myocardial revascularization in the elderly. Ann Intern Med 1994; 121:919-927.

Chapter 6

Stents, Also Known as Cosmetic Cardiology

As we discussed in an earlier chapter, coronary arteries treated by angioplasty will re-clog 40-50% of the time. In an effort to improve these statistics cardiologists often use a stent which is an expandable metal tube that is placed inside the artery which has just been opened or expanded by angioplasty. In order to get the stent into the blood vessel it is first collapsed to a very small size and then placed over an angioplasty balloon catheter and threaded through the blood vessels into the area of the blockage. When the doctor has found the proper location of the blockage, the balloon is inflated, the stent expands and is locked into place. The stent forms a rigid support to hold the artery open. Once the stent is inserted it remains there permanently. It holds open the blood vessel and improves blood flow to the heart and will usually relieve chest pain.

Stents are a fairly common procedure today and are used often. However, long term research on the effectiveness of stents is still lacking. Stents can sometimes be used as an alternative to coronary artery bypass surgery or in combination with angioplasty. Not all patients are candidates for angioplasty or a stent. If the size of the artery is too small or the location or size of the blockage is too big or covers too much of the length of the artery, it may not be possible to use angioplasty or stents. Using stents has been helpful in keeping the artery open for a longer period of time and decreasing the number of failures. It is important to note that even arteries with stents in them can still re-close. In order to try to prevent re-closure of a stent a doctor will place the patient on blood thinners and recommend the use of aspirin.

If you survive the surgery, the drugs used with stents could still harm you!

Because a stent is made of metal and is considered to be foreign, your body has a strong tendency to form a blood clot around the stent closing it off and of course defeating the reason it was put in. In order to keep a blood clot from forming in the stent your doctor will usually use a very strong class of medications called antiplatelet agents to prevent this process. One of several medications are usually used. The first is abciximab or ReoPro® (Eli Lilly & Co.), which is FDA approved to be used during and after angioplasty to prevent blood clotting. As you might expect this drug can lead to serious major bleeding complications! Approximately 21% of patients on this drug develop low blood pressure, 18% nausea, 11% vomiting, and almost 17% bleeding problems, some of them severe. And if these side effects don't get you, the price will. One course of treatment with ReoPro® is over $1,500. Tirofiban or Aggrastat® (Merck), is another anticlotting agent that is given by injection during angioplasty in order to prevent blood clots. The FDA requires blood tests every day while on this medication.

Another pharmaceutical, often used for stent placement and bypass surgery, is ticlopidine or Ticlid® (Roche Laboratories), a very powerful drug used to prevent blood clots. It is only approved by the FDA for use in patients at risk for blood clots that could cause a stroke. As of the writing of this book Ticlid® was *not FDA approved* to be used after any kind of heart surgery. Nevertheless, this dangerous medication is being used in many patients receiving stents and undergoing bypass surgery despite the fact that 60% of patients taking this medication will experience side effects. Ticlid® has the potential to be very dangerous and has what doctors call a "black box warning." In this warning the FDA requires the manufacturer to inform doctors and their patients that this medication can cause life threatening side effects including:

- low white blood count

- severely abnormal platelet count and
- bone marrow damage.

And this medication is so potentially dangerous that your doctor will need to do blood tests on you every two weeks for the first three months and for a while even after you stop the medication!

Plavix® or clopidogrel is sometimes used after stent surgery to prevent clotting of the stent. This medication like the others is not FDA approved for use during or after stent placement but nevertheless is commonly used.

You could be allergic to the stent.

Data recently published in the Lancet showed that metal allergy may contribute to stenosis in some patients who have had angioplasty with placement of stainless steel stents. These doctors demonstrated a link between allergy to metals like nickel and molybdenum and stenosis of the stent in the first six months after insertion.

How much do stents really help?

The following is an article published in the *American Journal of Cardiology* in 1988. Dr. Kornowski and his colleagues at the Washington Cardiology Center placed stents in 334 patients. The investigation revealed that there was a 7% failure rate in the hospital during stent placement. One percent of the patients died during stent placement and placement of the stent in some patients caused problems that were so severe they were immediately sent for emergency bypass surgery. When these patients were re-evaluated only one year later researchers found that 20% of the patients had developed new cardiac problems, 2.2% had died, 3.5% went on to have another heart attack and 11% of them required repeat surgery. The grand total of failures and complications in this study approaches almost 44%. The *American Journal of Cardiology* in 1999 published a study where they looked at patients that had undergone stents. They followed up the patients one year later and discovered that 23% of patients with stents had either died, suffered a repeat heart attack, undergone repeat angioplasty or needed coronary artery bypass surgery.

Pick one, stents or angioplasty.

Another study comparing stent placement and balloon angioplasty in the treatment of coronary artery disease was published in the *New England Journal of Medicine* in 1994 and was done at the Jefferson Medical College in Philadelphia, Pennsylvania. Researchers compared patients with stents to those without stents for six months following their procedure. They discovered that 20% of patients with stents and 24% of patients without stents had at least one of the following events occur:

- death
- myocardial infarction
- coronary artery bypass surgery
- vessel closure
- clotting of the stent and/or repeat angioplasty.

Unfortunately, the researchers only followed these patients for six months.

Also in 1998, a comparison study was done at Emory University. The researchers looked at a national registry of patients that had undergone angioplasty or treatment with new devices such as stents. The authors compared patients in the registry that had had balloon angioplasty with those treated with the newer technology such as stents. The researchers concluded, "this comparative study found no overall superiority of these newer devices in terms of patient survival." In other words at the end of the comparison period there was no difference in survival between the patient that had had balloon angioplasty compared with those that had stent placement.

Technology Junkies.

Although Eric Topol, M.D. from the Cleveland Clinic Foundation states that stents are one of the most important advances in cardiology in the last ten years he also voices concern that many cardiologists are "medical-technological junkies" that are "gorging on stents." To make matters worse manufacturers of stents are gouging the patient by charging an excessive mark up on stents, a reported profit margin of almost 90%! In the official journal of the American Heart Association, *Circulation*, Dr. Topol introduces the term "oculostenotic reflex" (oculo means eye, stenotic means blockage) to describe the "irresistible temptation among some invasive cardiologist to perform angioplasty" on any blockage they see regardless of whether the blockage is causing symptoms or not. Later in the same article the term "coronary cosmetology" is mentioned suggesting at times a cardiologist will place a stent in a narrowed artery simply to improve the appearance of the vessel on x-ray.

Heart laser surgery, another high tech treatment that doesn't work.

In order to perform transmyocardial laser revascularization the surgeon exposes the heart through an incision that cuts through the side of the chest. With the heart thus exposed, a laser is placed against the outside of the heart and anywhere from 10 to 50 holes or channels are burned into the heart. The prevailing theory is that these artificially created channels allow blood to circulate to the heart muscle.

There are several problems to consider when contemplating laser surgery for angina.

Unlike External CounterPulsation where blinded studies have been completed, no blinded studies have been done with this kind of heart laser surgery. There is a great bias among the general public that laser surgery is some kind of miracle. This kind of bias can make patients think that they got better when they really did not. Scientists call this a placebo effect. A blinded study is designed to eliminate this bias.

The suspicion that this just might be a placebo effect is supported by the fact that none of the patients showed better functioning of the heart after laser surgery. Just as significant is the fact that the great majority of patients studied after laser surgery did not show improved blood flow to the heart.

Patients did say that they had less chest pain after the laser surgery. Doctors critical of this therapy believe that the decreased chest pain is due to the fact that many of the nerves in the heart are destroyed during the intensive lasering process. This could explain why patients felt better while at the same time not showing any improved functioning of the heart muscle.

Laser surgery has a high rate of complications. A review of the current research shows that anywhere from 32 to 68% of patients that underwent laser treatment had side effects, which ranged from heart attacks to heart failure and infection.

This invasive laser procedure is not inexpensive. It requires a surgeon, hospital operating room, expensive laser equipment, and an extended hospital stay for recovery.

For patients with heart disease that cannot be repaired with surgery or angioplasty, there are other options besides dangerous laser therapy. L. David Hillis M.D., from the University of Texas Southwestern Medical Center, believes that External CounterPulsation is a much better choice for patients than laser therapy because it is more effective and much safer.

Fortunately today you have another choice. Now for the first time there is a proven, drug free, surgery free alternative, External CounterPulsation! Ask your doctor if you are a candidate for External CounterPulsation. You may not need to undergo repeated angioplasties, multiple stent surgeries and take dangerous drugs.

References:
Am J Cardiol 1998;82:1163-1167.

Kornowski R, Mehran R, Satler LF, et al. Procedural results and late clinical outcomes following multivesselcoronary stenting. J Am Coll Cardiol 1999 Feb;33(2):420-426.

Fischman DL, Leon MB, Baim DS, et al. A randomized comparison of coronary-stent placement and balloon angioplasty in the treatment of coronary artery disease. Stent Restenosis Study Investigators. N Engl J Med 1994 Aug 25;331(8):496-501.

King SB 3rd, Yeh W, Holubkov R, et al. Balloon angioplasty versus new device intervention: clinical outcomes. A comparison of the NHLBI PTCA and NACI registries. J Am Coll Cardiol 1998 Mar 1;31(3):558-566.

Topol EJ. Coronary-artery stents--gauging, gorging, and gouging. N Engl J Med 1998 Dec 3;339(23):1702-1704.

Topol EJ, Nissen SE. Our preoccupation with coronary luminology. The dissociation between clinical and angiographic findings in ischemic heart disease. Circulation 1995 Oct 15;92(8):2333-2342.

Lange RA, Hillis LD. Transmyocardial laser revascularization. N Engl J Med. 1999 Sep 30;341(14):1075-6.

Koster R, Vieluf D, Kiehn M, Sommerauer M, Kahler J, Baldus S, Meinertz T, Hamm CW. Nickel and molybdenum contact allergies in patients with coronary in-stent restenosis. Lancet. 2000;356(9245):1895-7.

Chapter 7

Coronary Artery Bypass Grafting, Seduced by Technology

Coronary Artery Bypass Grafting
(CABG, pronounced "cabbage")

What is Coronary Bypass Surgery?

Coronary artery bypass surgery is a heart operation that uses blood vessels from the legs or arms called veins, or blood vessels from the chest called arteries to go around or bypass clogged coronary arteries. In order for the doctors to get into your chest they will have to saw through your sternum or breastbone. The entire procedure is done under anesthesia and can take 3 to 6 hours. While this is being done you are kept alive by a mechanical device called a heart lung machine which breathes for you and artificially circulates your blood. Afterwards you will spend several days in the Intensive Care Unit. You will have more tubes, wires and needles put in or on your body than you ever thought possible. You will have a tube in your throat that is connected to a ventilator for the first 24 hours in order to help you breathe. Family coming to visit bypass patients the first day after surgery are usually shocked and frightened to see a loved one in such a situation. Bypass patients deserve flowers, lots of flowers.

A review of the CABG literature, the last 21 years.

In 1978 the *New England Journal of Medicine* published an article looking at the long-term fate of coronary artery bypass grafts. The conclusion, "...although most patients improved symptomatically after operation, symptomatic deterioration is common in the succeeding years." Sixty-eight percent of the patients had a return of cardiac symptoms within five years after bypass surgery.

Flunked the treadmill? Don't sign up for surgery yet!

Doctor Graboys along with other researchers published a 1981 article in the *New England Journal of Medicine* in which they studied coronary artery disease patients with severe ECG changes called ST segment depression that occurred during treadmill exercising testing. Usually patients with this kind of severe ECG change are immediately scheduled for surgery. What would happen if these patients were treated medically instead of surgically? The results were surprising. Doctor Graboys discovered that flunking the treadmill did not mean that surgery was always absolutely necessary. The outcome was summarized as follows: "We conclude that such ST depression is not associated with a poor prognosis. There is rarely a need to resort to cardiac surgery; medical management is highly successful and associated with a low mortality."

Not everyone with mild angina or a previous heart attack needs surgery.

A group of 780 heart disease patients were divided with one half treated only with medication and the other half treated with coronary artery bypass surgery. After five years, 82% of the medically treated patients and 83% of the surgically treated patients were alive and free of heart attacks. The conclusion of this article published in 1984 was as follows, "As compared with medical therapy, coronary artery bypass surgery appears neither to prolong life nor to prevent myocardial infarction in patients who have mild angina or are asymptomatic after infarction."

Bypassed coronary blood vessels clog ten times faster!

In 1984 the prestigious *New England Journal of Medicine* published a study which showed that when coronary vessels with less than 50% blockage are bypassed, they clog up ten times faster than they normally would! The conclusion of the study was that minimally diseased coronary arteries should not be bypassed at all. Bypass surgery may therefore result in more bypass surgery.

Who does benefit from bypass surgery?

These physicians authored an article in the *American Journal of Cardiology* which discovered after ten years of study that coronary artery bypass graft or CABG, "should probably remain limited to patients with incapacitating anginal symptoms or to those with severe lesions for whom surgery might enhance long-term survival, such as patients with severe left main coronary artery disease and three vessel coronary artery disease." (Please refer to heart diagram in Chapter 9.)

So, is your heart disease bad enough for bypass surgery?

An 11-year Veterans Administration study compared mortality for medical versus surgical treatments for stable angina. What they found was two different risk groups. After 11 years 43% of the low risk medically treated patients died while 42% of the low risk surgically treated patients died. However, the 11 year death rate for the high risk surgically treated patients was 46% while the high risk medically treated patients had an 11 year death rate of 76%. It is quite clear from this study that surgery only helped the high-risk patients.

Another similar study published in the *New England Journal of Medicine* in 1985 compared coronary artery bypass surgery with medical therapy for patients 65 years of age or older. This study was from the Coronary Artery Surgery Study registry, also known as CASS. Again these researchers found that surgical benefit was greatest in the high-risk patients with the poorest prognosis. In the low risk patients with mild angina and good functioning ventricles with no left main coronary artery disease, there was no survival difference between those treated with only medicines and those treated with surgery.

You need a second opinion! You need a second opinion!

In 1987 the *Journal of the American Medical Association* published a study looking at the usefulness of obtaining second opinions before allowing patients to undergo bypass surgery.

Researchers evaluated 88 patients with an average age of 59 years who were seen for a second opinion as to whether these patients really needed coronary artery bypass graft surgery. All of the patients had an angiogram which showed significant multiple vessel coronary artery disease in 72% of them while the remaining 28% had single vessel disease involving only the left anterior descending coronary artery. The doctors then recommended that 84% of the patients *not* undergo bypass surgery at that time! When complete this study revealed that second opinions could safely reduce the need for coronary artery bypass graft operations in selected patients by as much as 50%!

Want more recent proof?

The previous study is further supported by an article looking at the appropriateness of performing coronary artery bypass surgery and was done through the UCLA Center for Health Sciences. Published in 1988 in the *Journal of the American Medical Association*, researchers reviewed several hospitals to determine the appropriateness of previously performed coronary artery bypass surgery. Several hundred cases over a period of a few years were reviewed. What they discovered was that 56% of the surgeries were performed for appropriate reasons. However, 44% of the coronary artery bypass surgeries were performed for inappropriate or equivocal reasons! Their conclusion was that eliminating inappropriate bypass surgery might lead to reductions in health care spending and to better patient outcomes.

Will your brain survive bypass surgery?

This study published in the journal *Stroke* reviewed approximately 300 patients that had undergone coronary artery bypass surgery for brain injury: Sixty-one percent had neurological complications, 79% had neuropsychological complications and 24% had severe intellectual dysfunction. The researchers speculated that the brain injury appeared to have resulted from use of the heart lung bypass machine while surgery was being performed.

Survival after a heart attack is worse when patients have had previous coronary artery bypass surgery.

This very interesting five year study is from the Montreal Heart Institute in Quebec, Canada. Two very similar groups of heart attack patients with the same amount of coronary artery disease were studied with the only difference being that one group had previous bypass surgery while the other did not. Over a period of five years, it was discovered that the bypass patients had 74% more repeat heart attacks, 27% more admissions to the hospital for unstable angina, 20% more deaths and 70% more angioplasties and bypasses than the similar group of heart attack patients that had never had bypass surgery.

The following article doesn't even need to be discussed, we can learn a lot just from the title. Published in *Circulation,* the title of the article is "Coronary Artery Bypass Grafting For The Third Time or More. Results of 150 Cases". This article reviewed patients who had undergone three, four and even five separate coronary bypass surgeries.

What happens to patients who refuse coronary artery bypass surgery?

One hundred fifty patients, average age of 57, who refused to have bypass surgery were followed for eight years. The results were published in the 1990 *American Journal of Cardiology.* Eight percent of these patients had single vessel coronary artery disease, and 92% had multiple vessel coronary artery disease. A co-author of the paper, Doctor Hueb discovered that medical treatment in patients with advanced coronary artery disease but with good pumping function of the heart muscle had good survival and remission of symptoms without the surgery.

Know your ejection fraction.

In order to understand what follows you have to know what

ejection fraction means. Ejection fraction simply refers to the efficiency with which the heart is able to pump. For example, if your heart has 100 ml of blood in it and it pumps out 50 ml then the ejection fraction is 50%.

Stanford University researchers followed seven hundred eighty patients from the Coronary Artery Surgery Study that were divided into either a coronary surgery group or a medical therapy group. After ten years, there was no difference in survival. Eighty percent of both the medical and surgical groups were still alive. However, the researchers did go on to say that survival was somewhat better when surgery was performed on those heart patients with weak pumps that had an ejection fraction less than 50%. Patients with a strong heart pump that had an ejection fraction of more than 50% did better without surgery.

Benefits of bypass surgery transient.

Another very engaging study published in *Circulation* was titled "18 Year Follow Up In The Veterans Affairs Cooperative Study of Coronary Artery Bypass Surgery For Stable Angina. The VA Coronary Artery Bypass Surgery Cooperative Study Group." In this investigation, 686 stable angina patients were studied for 18 years. The patients were randomly assigned to either surgical or medical therapy. The conclusions of this long-term extensive study were as follows: "The benefits of coronary artery bypass surgery on survival, symptoms, and the post infarction mortality were transient and lasted fewer than 11 years." The article went on to say that low risk patients who had a good prognosis derived absolutely no survival benefit from surgery at any time during this study. Regardless of risk, these researchers found that surgery did not reduce the incidence of heart attacks in these patients or reduce the number of deaths.

Bypass surgery does not improve survival.

In 1998 the *American Journal of Cardiology* published a 22

year follow up of the VA Cooperative study of Coronary Artery Bypass Surgery. What these researchers observed is similar to what was found earlier in the 18 year study. Strong evidence from this 22-year study revealed that initial bypass surgery did not improve survival for patients that were at low risk and it did not reduce the risk of having a heart attack. Although the researchers felt there was some early benefit to the high-risk heart patients having surgery, long-term survival rates were similar in both the surgical and medical treatment groups. They also noted that twice as many bypass procedures were performed in the group assigned to surgery without these patients benefiting from living longer or experiencing greater improvement of symptoms.

The National Medicare Experience after bypass surgery.

Any Medicare patient contemplating bypass surgery should be aware of the following research completed by Dr. Eric Peterson and his associates at Duke University Medical Center. Unfortunately elderly patients are rarely quoted accurate figures. Please remember that this study looks only at the death rate after successful bypass surgery. If strokes, kidney failure, infections and depression are also taken into account the rate of morbidity and mortality could easily exceed 50%. The statistics cited below are reality. Please choose treatment for your heart disease carefully. The cure may be more dangerous than your disease. If, in the unusual event that ECP and medication fails, you can always attempt bypass surgery later.

The National Medicare Experience Death After Bypass Surgery in 357,885 Patients		
Ages	30 Day % death rate	1 Year % death rate
65-69	4.3	8.0
70-74	5.7	10.9
75-79	7.4	14.2
Greater than 80	10.6	19.5

How well do women do with bypass surgery?

If you are a woman scheduled for bypass surgery, watch out! In this 1993 study completed at University of Southern California, it was found that women undergoing bypass surgery had a 42% higher mortality than men. And a 1999 article written by Dr. Charles Hogue and colleagues from the Washington School of Medicine revealed even worse statistics. This article published in *Circulation* revealed that the in-hospital death after heart surgery was 86% higher for women than for men or almost double the men's death rate. Why is this you ask? Research published in *Circulation* observed that women with a smaller body frame and stature were at increased risk for in-hospital death from coronary artery bypass graft surgery. They discovered when small vessels were bypassed that the patient was ten times more likely to die than a patient with larger blood vessels undergoing bypass. The doctors concluded that these findings supported the fact that women with smaller coronary arteries and smaller people in general have higher in-hospital mortality.

Minorities do not do well with bypass surgery either.

In 1996 the *Archives of Internal Medicine* published a study discussing the adverse outcome blacks have in the five years following coronary artery bypass surgery. The conclusion of this study was "In this group of predominantly medically insured patients undergoing coronary artery bypass surgery the risk of death in blacks at five years was twice that of whites."

Most bypass surgeries and angioplasties can be postponed indefinitely.
In the 1998 December issue of the *U.S. News & World Report* Thomas B. Graboys, M.D., Associate Clinical Professor of Medicine, Harvard Medical School stated that the majority of coronary artery disease patients can be successfully treated without such invasive procedures as bypass surgery and angioplasty. He explained that the majority of research from Harvard and other medical institutions strongly suggest that coronary artery disease patients treated with medications do just as well if not better than those patients who undergo invasive procedures. Dr. Graboys elaborated stating that in his practice 800 patients whose average age was 71, when treated medically, had a lower mortality than those treated with surgery. He clarified this by going on to state that some patients clearly do need bypass surgery but "….two thirds of all bypass surgery and angioplasty can be *safely* deferred or postponed indefinitely." Graboys concluded: "Regrettably, the rush to invasive procedures is fueled by nonclinical factors, profit among them."

So why don't bypass surgery patients do all that much better?
1. Since coronary artery bypass surgery treats only the symptoms without treating the cause, angina and heart attacks will continue to recur and worsen.
2. Bypass surgery treats heart disease as a simple plumbing problem which it obviously is not. Heart disease is a complex biochemical problem, which needs comprehensive medical and nutritional treatment for best results.
3. Just because a blockage is there doesn't mean it has to be

surgically corrected. Unstable blockages that cause heart attacks are often small and do not appear significant on an angiogram. Large blockages that look dangerous may not be dangerous because they are not necessarily unstable. Simply stated 90% blockages usually cause angina. It is blockages that are smaller than 70% that are responsible for the majority of heart attacks. This may seem to go against common sense but it is a proven fact.

4. Women and small-framed people often have blood vessels too small to safely bypass or angioplasty.

5. Over two thirds of bypass surgeries are probably not necessary. Get a second opinion. Know your ejection fraction, if it is over 50% think twice about any type of surgery.

If all you have is a hammer, then everything gets treated like a nail.

You can probably postpone bypass surgery indefinitely if:

- You are a candidate for External CounterPulsation! In fact **ECP** is making **CABG** stand for **C**an **A**void **B**ypass **G**rafting

- A treadmill test shows that you do not have abnormal heart rhythms that develop from exercise

- You respond well to medications and are stable using them.

Physicians and patients alike are finding the benefits from ECP to be dramatic. As a result ECP is rapidly becoming known as the only FDA-cleared treatment that can do a **NCAB** or **N**atural **C**oronary **A**rtery **B**ypass.

References:
Seides SF, Borer JS, Kent KM, et al. Long-term anatomic fate of coronary-artery bypass grafts and functional status of patients five years after operation. N Engl J Med 1978 Jun 1;298(22):1213-1217.

Podrid PJ, Graboys TB, Lown B. Prognosis of medically treated patients with coronary-artery disease with profound ST-segment depression during exercise testing. N Engl J Med 1981 Nov 5;305(19):1111-1116.

Myocardial infarction and mortality in the coronary artery surgery study (CASS) randomized trial. N Engl J Med 1984 Mar 22;310(12):750-758.

Cashin WL, Sanmarco ME, Nessim SA, et al. Accelerated progression of atherosclerosis in coronary vessels with minimal lesions that are bypassed. N Engl J Med 1984 Sep 27;311(13):824-828.

Bourassa MG, Enjalbert M, Campeau L, et al. Progression of atherosclerosis in coronary arteries and bypass grafts: ten years later. Am J Cardiol 1984 Jun 15;53(12):102C-107C.

Long-term mortality and morbidity results of the Veterans Administration randomized trial of coronary artery bypass surgery. Circulation 1985 Dec;72(6 Pt 2):V84-89.

Comparison of coronary artery bypass surgery and medical therapy in patients 65 years of age or older. A nonrandomized study from the Coronary Artery Surgery Study (CASS) registry. New Engl J Med 1985 Jul 25;313(4):217-24.

Graboys TB, Headley A, Lown B, et al. Results of a second-opinion program for coronary artery bypass graft surgery. JAMA 1987 Sep 25;258(12):1611-1614.

Shaw PJ, Bates D, Cartlidge NE, et al. Neurologic and neuropsychological morbidity following major surgery: comparison of coronary artery bypass and peripheral vascular surgery. Stroke 1987 Jul-Aug;18(4):700-707.

Wiseman A, Waters DD, Walling A, et al. Long-term prognosis after myocardial infarction in patients with previous coronary artery bypass surgery. J Am Coll Cardiol 1988 Oct;12(4):873-880.

Winslow CM, Kosecoff JB, Chassin M, et al. The appropriateness of performing coronary artery bypass surgery. JAMA 1988 Jul 22-29;260(4):505-509.

Brenowitz JB, Johnson WD, Kayser KL, et al. Coronary artery bypass grafting for the third time or more. Results of 150 consecutive cases. Circulation 1988 Sep;78(3 Pt 2):I166-170.

Hueb W, Bellotti G, Ramires JA, et al. Two- to eight-year survival rates in patients who refused coronary artery bypass grafting. Am J Cardiol 1989 Jan 15;63(3):155-159.

Alderman EL, Bourassa MG, Cohen LS, et al. Ten-year follow-up of survival and myocardial infarction in the randomized Coronary Artery Surgery Study. Circulation 1990 Nov;82(5):1629-1646.

Eighteen-year follow-up in the Veterans Affairs Cooperative Study of Coronary Artery Bypass. Surgery for stable angina. The VA Coronary Artery Bypass Surgery Cooperative Study Group. Cooperative Studies Program, VA Medical Center, West Haven, Conn 06516. Circulation 1992 Jul;86(1):121-130.

Rahimtoola SH, Bennett AJ, Grunkemeier GL, et al. Survival at 15 to 18 years after coronary bypass surgery for angina in women. Circulation 1993 Nov;88(5 Pt 2):II71-178.

Gray RJ, Nessim S, Khan SS, et al. Arch Intern Med 1996 Apr 8;156(7):769-773 Adverse 5-year outcome after coronary artery bypass surgery in blacks.

O'Connor NJ, Morton JR, Birkmeyer JD, et al. Effect of coronary artery diameter in patients undergoing coronary bypass surgery. Circulation 1996 Feb 15;93(4):652-655.

Forrester JS, Shah PK. Lipid lowering versus revascularization: an idea whose time (for testing) has come. Circulation 1997 Aug 1996(4):1360-1362.

Peduzzi P, Kamina A, Detre K. Twenty-two-year follow-up in the VA Cooperative Study of Coronary Artery Bypass Surgery for Stable Angina. Am J Cardiol 1998 Jun 15;81(12):1393-1399.

Hogue C, et al. Women at higher risk of stroke after cardiac surgery than men. Circulation 1999;100;642-647.

Peterson ED, Jollis JG, Bebchuk JD, et al. Changes in mortality after myocardial revascularization in the elderly. Ann Intern Med 1994; 121:919-927.

Chapter 8

Discovery of External CounterPulsation

1953

In 1953 Kantrowitz and Kantrowitz discovered that the coronary blood flow of animals could be increased by up to 40% if the blood pressure during diastole (the resting phase) was increased. Later on in 1968 Kantrowitz developed an internal system which consisted of a balloon pump attached to a long wire called a catheter, inserted into the femoral artery and then threaded into the aorta near the heart. Once in place, this internal aortic balloon pump was used to assist cardiac blood flow in patients undergoing surgery or with weak hearts. The way this internal pump works to help the heart is similar in many ways to the External CounterPulsation devices now in use. Today cardiac surgeons nationwide use a more modern version of Dr. Kantrowitz's device.

1962

In 1962, Harry S. Soroff, M.D. and colleagues introduced the term "counterpulsation." Soroff demonstrated that the heart worked more efficiently when "counter pulsation" was implemented during diastole (the resting phase of the heart.) A catheter was inserted into the femoral artery in the leg, which contained a balloon device. The balloon was quickly inflated during diastole, causing blood to be pumped back to the heart. The balloon was then immediately deflated prior to the beginning of the next heartbeat. Although this procedure did in fact prove the soundness of Soroff's theory, it was not a comfortable procedure for the patient.

A few years later, Birtwell, Dennis and Giron developed an improved External CounterPulsation device, which was hydraulically activated. Their rendition consisted of rigid pipes that were placed around the legs of the patient. Inside these pipes were balloons that fit around the legs. These balloons could be filled with water (much like a blood pressure cuff fills with air) to compress the patient's legs. During diastole the balloons inside the pipes filled with water and squeezed the legs thereby pushing the blood in the legs back up to the heart. Birtwell, Dennis and Giron documented that this therapy was effective in improving the survival rate following heart attacks.

At about this same time, another researcher successfully accomplished counterpulsation using a pilot's G-suit. G forces generated during combat flying force blood out of the brain into the legs, which can make a pilot pass out. A G-suit is simply a tight fitting pair of pants that can be inflated squeezing the blood out of the legs back into the chest, heart and brain. It is typically worn by fighter pilots in order to keep them from passing out during high speed maneuvers. Osborn's findings were good, but his procedures were too uncomfortable for the patient and were discontinued.

1970

By the 1970's External CounterPulsation devices were used to treat angina, again with favorable results. In fact the improved circulation to the heart was so significant it could be demonstrated on before and after angiograms.

Z.S. Zheng, a Chinese physician developed an improved version of the ECP device in the 1980's which utilized five cuffs, two on each leg and one buttock cuff. These cuffs were sequentially inflated from the calf to the thigh to the buttock. Zheng treated a group of 200 chronic angina patients with his ECP device and was able to demonstrate that 97% of the patients exhibited prolonged symptomatic improvement. Zheng also noticed that these patients consistently exhibited an increased ability to exercise. This study, along with others and further technological improvements of ECP has led to the wide spread use and acceptance of ECP in China. In the

United States ECP is just beginning to be accepted. We have a long way to go to catch up with the 1500 ECP units being used in China. It may be that ECP was more readily embraced in China because there is no billion-dollar heart industry.

1980

In 1980 the *American Journal of Cardiology* published a 25 institution multi-center study in which 258 acute heart attack patients were given External CounterPulsation. The patients receiving ECP therapy had over a 50% decrease in death rate compared to those patients who did not receive External CounterPulsation. In 1987 Cardiomedics, based in California, became the first US company to receive marketing clearance from the FDA for its External CounterPulsation system for angina. Cardiomedics provides CardiAssist™ External CounterPulsation. Vasomedical received their FDA clearance for EECP® in 1995.

References:
Kantrowitz A, Kantrowitz A. Experimental augmentation of coronary flow by retardation of arterial pressure pulse. Surgery. 1953;34:678-687.

Soroff SJ, Britwell WC, Levine HS, et al. Effect of counterpulsation upon myocardial oxygen consumption and heart work. Surg Forum Am Coll of Surgery. 1962;13:174.

Birtwell WC, Giron F, Soroff HS, et al. Support of systemic circulation and left ventricular assist by synchronous pulsation of extramural pressure. Trans Am Soc Artif Intern Organs. 1965;11:43-52.

Osborn JJ, Russi M, Salel A, et al. Circulatory assistance by external pulsed pressures. Am J Med Electronics. 1964;iii:87-90

Amsterdam, EM, Banas J, Criley JM, et al. Clinical Assessment of External Pressure Circulatory Assistance in Acute Myocardial Infarction. Report of a Cooperative Clinical Trial. Am. J. Cardiology. 45:349-56, 1980

Zheng Zs, Li TM, Kambic H, et al. Sequential external counterpulsation (SECP) in China. Trans Am Soc Artif Intern Organs. 1983;29:599-603

Chapter 9
External CounterPulsation
How To Do a
Natural Coronary Artery Bypass
(aka: Everything you have always wanted
to know about the heart.)

In order to understand how sequential enhanced External CounterPulsation or ECP works, it's important to understand a little bit about the circulatory system. (Note: ECP is also referred to as E^2CP, SECP, doubleE-CP, Enhanced External CounterPulsation CardiAssist™ by Cardiomedics or EECP® by Vasomedical.)

The normal heart is slightly larger than your fist and is shaped nothing like the box of candy you got for Valentine's Day but more so like a lopsided grapefruit. We have all heard the infamous beat of the heart either through a doctor's stethoscope, a fetal monitor, or simply by resting our head on the chest of a wife or husband. We have heard the "lub-dub, lub-dub" of a heart so many times, but most likely took those sounds for granted.

The heart is a muscle by definition and a pump by design. Each minute the average heart beats (or "contracts") 72 times and pumps one and a half gallons of blood. Each hour, the heart contracts 4320 times and pumps 84 gallons of blood. Each moment of contraction (lub-dub) lasts less than approximately 0.40 seconds (less than one-half of a second) and is called "systole".

Following each contraction the heart "rests" (lub-dub, rest, lub-dub, rest). Each moment of "rest" lasts approximately 0.43 seconds and is called "diastole." When your blood pressure is taken, the doctor obtains two numbers or "readings." For example, if your blood pressure is 120/80, the 120 is the systolic pressure (or contracting pressure of your heart) and the 80 is the diastolic pressure (or resting pressure of your heart.)

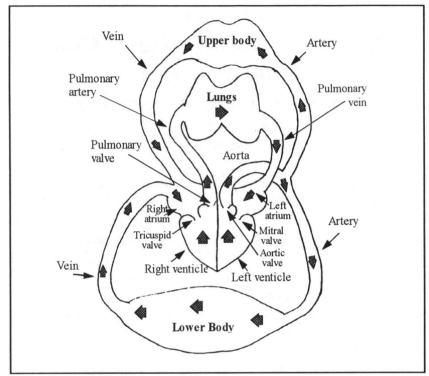

Figure 1. Circulation of blood through the heart and body

    The heart has four sections or "chambers." (See Fig. 1) On the right, is the "right atrium" and the "right ventricle." These two chambers interact with the lungs. On the left side of the heart is the "left atrium" and the "left ventricle." The walls of the left side of the heart are approximately three times thicker than those of the right because the left side of the heart is responsible for pumping blood to the entire body.

    Our bodies are in constant need of nourishment and just like an automobile we require fuel and oxygen to function. Blood supplies the fuel and oxygen that our bodies need and travels to every organ via vessels called "arteries." One of the most critical components carried in blood is oxygen. If you have ever held your breath for any significant length of time you know how desperately your body needs oxygen.

Blood that is carrying oxygen (also called "oxygenated blood"), is bright red in color and usually travels in arteries. The only exception to this is the pulmonary vein which carries oxygenated blood to the heart. Likewise the pulmonary artery is the only artery that carries unoxygenated blood. After this oxygenated blood is delivered to the cells of our body the oxygen is removed and the blood becomes bluish in color. It is returned to the right atrium in vessels called "veins." These veins are most often found along side the arteries and are connected with smaller vessels called "capillaries." Although not often thought of as an organ, all the blood vessels put together would weigh as much as the liver. If the inside lining of our blood vessels called the "endothelium" was laid out flat it would cover six tennis courts. Together with the heart, the arteries and veins work together to form the "circulatory system" of the body.

Even as you read this page, your heart is pumping blood. The right atrium is receiving bluish, oxygen depleted blood from all the veins in your body. The blood is filling up the right atrium and then is pumped into the right ventricle. From there, it is pumped into your lungs, where the waste gas (carbon dioxide) is removed and more oxygen is picked up by the blood. The oxygenated blood is now bright red again and is sent to the left atrium. After a moment there, it is pumped into the left ventricle and then out through the aorta and to your entire body once again.

But how does the heart receive nourishment and oxygen from the blood? Just as your body contains a sophisticated circulatory system, the heart itself has its own system of arteries, called the "coronary circulatory system." And, it is the condition of this particular system that is of the utmost importance to the functioning of the rest of your body.

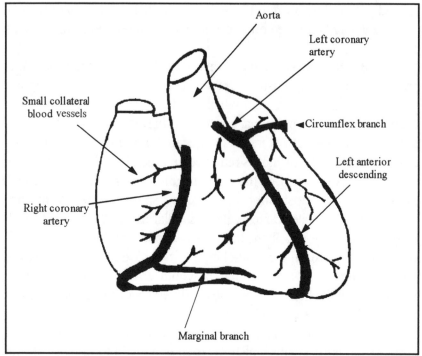

Figure 2. Coronary artery circulation of the heart

The heart receives its nutritive blood and oxygen supply from two main arteries and one branch: the right coronary artery and the left coronary artery. (See Fig. 2) The right coronary artery originates at the aorta and descends along the surface of the heart towards the right and supplies the right ventricle heart muscle with blood. The left coronary artery also originates at the aorta, but descends along the front surface of the heart. This artery supplies the left ventricle muscle with blood and is also known as the left anterior descending artery or "LAD." This LAD artery has a branch called the "left circumflex" artery which wraps around the surface to the back (or "posterior") of the heart.

These three arteries are the main vessels that supply blood to the heart. When a doctor says there is evidence of "triple vessel disease," it means that these three vessels show evidence of atherosclerosis or blockage.

It is important to note that the heart muscle can only receive its blood during "diastole" (the resting phase of the heart). All the other tissues in the body receive blood when the heart is pumping; not so with the heart itself. Blood is unable to enter the coronary arteries during "systole" (the pumping phase) when the heart is contracting, because the heart muscle is squeezing out blood so forcefully. However, when the heart is in its resting phase, the coronary arteries fill with oxygen enriched blood that nourishes the heart muscle.

Exercise and the heart.

When a person is at rest the amount of blood which flows through the coronary arteries measures just under a cup per minute. When a person is exercising, this amount may increase to five cups per minute. While most organs extract only 25% of the available oxygen from the blood, the heart extracts 75% of the oxygen even when a person is resting. Consequently, the only way the heart can receive extra oxygen during periods of exercise or increased demand is through increased blood flow. If this blood flow cannot be increased (due to blockages), then "angina" or a heart attack results.

"Angina pectoris" is merely the Latin term for "heart pain." Angina usually is felt beneath the upper sternum (breast bone) and may spread to the left arm or shoulder, the neck, jaw or the face. Most often, people experience angina when they exercise or are under increased stress. The pressure/pain sensation usually lasts only a few minutes, but in more severe or chronic cases the pressure may be constant.

Angina is usually treated with nitroglycerin, which causes a sudden dilation (widening) of veins throughout the body. The end result is that the amount of oxygen that the heart needs to function is reduced and in many patients there will be immediate relief of pain.

How ECP works.

At one time or another, everyone has blown up a balloon. Most of the balloons we have blown up over the years are the typical round ones, right? Well, have you ever blown up one of those long, skinny balloons? The ones that can be twisted and knotted and turned into poodles or dinosaurs?

Let's pretend you are holding one of these long, skinny balloons in your hands right now. You have the knotted end of the balloon in one hand and the other end of the balloon in the opposite hand. What would happen if you squeezed one of your hands around one end of the balloon? The air from that spot would be forced towards the other end of the balloon, right? The other end of the balloon would become slightly fatter. Well, this simple concept is the exact same principle used with ECP.

Earlier, we talked about how many times the heart beats each minute. We learned that the heart beats (systole) 72 times per minute and 4320 times per hour. We also learned that the heart "rested" (diastole) 4320 times per hour and that it was during these moments of "rest" that the heart itself obtained the blood it needs from the coronary arteries. Now, we will discover how ECP works during these systole and diastole cycles of the heart.

The External CounterPulsation units used today are somewhat larger and taller than a home desk. It operates on standard household electric current. Within the unit is a highly sophisticated computer microprocessor, a monitor, an electrocardiogram, an extremely sensitive pressure sensor, three hoses, five pressure cuffs and an air compressor.

Compressed air is held in pressure tanks and is available instantly on demand. While operating, the unit makes a sort of thumping, rushing air sound in exact synchrony with your heart rhythm. Each of the three hoses is connected to six pressure bladders sewn inside five cuffs. These five cuffs are placed on the patient as follows: one cuff at each calf, one cuff at each thigh and one large cuff: containing two air bladders at the buttocks. Two sensors are attached to the patient's fingers; one to measure pulse pressure tracings called plethysmography and one to measure blood oxygen levels. Three self adhesive ECG electrodes are placed on the patient's chest. All these readings are fed into the computer and analyzed to control the precise inflation of each of the cuffs at the exact moment the heart is in diastole.

The process of inflation begins at the calves, proceeds to the thighs, then the buttocks (see Fig. 3). The sequential inflation process of the five cuffs is in essence "milking" or massaging the blood from the calves up to the thighs, out of the buttocks and back up to the heart. This back flow of blood to the heart during diastole occurs in a matter of milliseconds. At the instant the computer determines that the heart is starting the next beat all five cuffs simultaneously and instantly deflates. This sudden deflation and the relative lack of blood in the legs creates somewhat of a "vacuum" which makes it much easier now for the heart to pump out the next volume of blood. ECP is thereby able to improve the pumping efficiency and output of the heart as well as provide more blood to the oxygen-starved areas of the heart.

What occurs during ECP treatment is truly amazing. When the blood is forced back into the coronary arteries during diastole these arteries are gently stretched, just like when you squeeze a long balloon. This abrupt pulse of blood through the coronary arteries causes the expansion of additional tiny collateral arteries, which normally are not functional. These smaller arteries or "collateral blood vessels," are found in everyone's heart but are often too small to be seen by the naked eye.

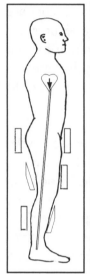
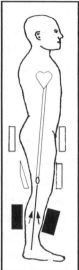
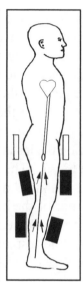
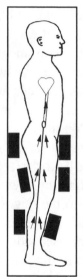
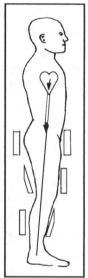

End of systole when the heart is fully contracted and a "pulse" has been pumped to the body.

The heart is now "resting" in diastole and CounterPulsation begins with inflation of the right and left calf cuffs.

Just milliseconds later the next two thigh cuffs inflate.

And just fractions of a second later the buttocks cuff inflates causing a surge of blood back to the heart and the entire upper body. Now instead of your organs getting 72 pulses of blood per minute they are getting 144. This extra blood benefits not only the heart but also the kidneys, reproductive organs, liver, eyes, and brain. Counterpulsation is complete.

The on board computer senses that the heart is beginning to start systole or contract and all five pressures cuffs immediately and instantly deflate. Since the leg arteries are empty they will fill very easily. Now the heart will not have to work nearly as hard pumping blood. This sequence of inflation and deflation is then repeated up to 4,300 times per hour.

Figure 3. Sequential External CounterPulsation.

The collateral vessels located on the surface of the heart are usually quite small under normal conditions. However, with the proper stimulation they have the potential to grow and enlarge delivering more blood to the heart. When the large coronary arteries surrounding the heart become clogged or blocked, the body can respond under the right conditions by developing alternate routes or detours around the blockages. The growth of these collateral vessels is a natural and beneficial response and is the body's attempt to protect the heart muscle from tissue death when the normal blood supply is cut off. Unfortunately, the body is seldom able to completely restore sufficient blood flow to the heart on its own. As you can imagine the enlargement of collateral vessels would be very helpful in protecting you from a heart attack when the normal blood supply is cut off due to a blockage.

As we discussed earlier, an angioplasty is a procedure where the doctor inserts a ballooning device into the coronary arteries, which causes the arteries to "expand" or stretch. ECP also causes the coronary arteries to expand. But with ECP the stretching is much more controlled, much more natural, and obviously does not require the use of a six foot catheter inserted through your groin or arm and snaked up to your heart.

With ECP, the coronary blood vessels are gently stretched over 4,000 times in a one hour treatment by the use of the body's own blood. During these thousands of gentle surges of blood, new vessels are slowly formed around the heart ready to supply much needed oxygen and nutrients. In the course of 35 one-hour treatments (the recommended initial treatment protocol) over 150,000 counter pulses of blood gently encourage the growth and expansion of new collateral blood vessels. Not only does the heart benefit from this additional blood flow but so do the kidneys, reproductive organs, intestines, lungs, eyes and brain. This may explain why patients who receive ECP often notice improvement in other areas besides the heart.

It is also hypothesized that this repeated gentle surge of blood acts as a mechanical stress (shear stress) leading to the release of blood vessel growth factors and consequently the development and enlargement of new blood vessels. Scientists have recently discovered that the use of ECP leads to an increase of a substance called "vascular endothelial growth factor" or "VEGF." This powerful blood vessel growth factor contributes to the growth and enlargement of new arteries, much like the hormones of puberty lead to the growth and enlargement of the different male and female body parts.

Think of ECP as an external "second heart" temporarily "attached" to your legs assisting your own heart, between beats. (Hence the name CardiAssist™ by Cardiomedics.) Now instead of your organs getting 72 pulses of blood per minute they are getting 144 pulses per minute. In many ways ECP provides the benefits of more blood flow like exercise does. However, unlike exercise, this increased blood flow occurs without the heart having to pump harder or faster. In fact the heart has actually been found to work more efficiently and with less effort while undergoing ECP. What could be safer than using ECP to harness the body's own healing processes for a completely natural coronary artery bypass?

References:
Soran O, Crawford LE, Schneider VM, et al. Enhanced external counterpulsation in the management of patients with cardiovascular disease. Clin Cardiol 1999 Mar;22(3):173-178.

Chapter 10
A New Dawn in Cardiology, Scientific Articles about External CounterPulsation.

External CounterPulsation is very effective.

Over the past several years many doctors, researchers and universities have treated cardiac patients with ECP and have documented the effectiveness of the treatment. From Boston to San Francisco patients are being helped and healed by ECP.

In 1992, Dr. Lawson and colleagues published an article in the *American Journal of Cardiology* documenting the use of ECP in 18 chronic angina patients. Prior to ECP every one of these patients were taking maximum doses of medication including nitroglycerin, beta-blockers and/or calcium channel blockers. At the time these patients started the External CounterPulsation they were having incapacitating angina despite maximum drug therapy! Eight of the eighteen patients alone accounted for nineteen previous heart surgeries consisting of either angioplasty or bypass surgery or both. Seven of the patients had had a total of fourteen heart attacks.

After treatment with ECP all 18 patients had a substantial improvement in angina and 16 had complete relief from angina during their usual activities of daily living. Many were able to reduce their medications. Fourteen patients had either complete or partial improvement in circulation according to the thallium stress testing performed after External CounterPulsation. Just 35 one-hour ECP treatment sessions were needed to obtain these exceptional results. These results are even more impressive when you consider that these patients already had tried the best that modern medicine could offer including drugs and surgery and they still had incapacitating angina. It wasn't until they completed a course of External CounterPulsation that significant lasting relief was obtained.

This man had angina, severe angina.

In 1997, *Clinical Cardiology* published a case study about a 58-year-old man with extensive triple vessel disease and severe angina. This gentleman had undergone 2 bypass operations and 18 angioplasties in a 3 year period. After 120 sessions of ECP, he was able to discontinue his nitroglycerin and demonstrated an improved ability to walk. Thallium stress testing revealed a total clearing of all of his previous circulation defects. Follow up office visits revealed that he remained asymptomatic for more than 3 years.

More difficult patients.

Doctor Strobeck reported in the *Journal of Cardiovascular Management* on two cardiac patients and their response to External CounterPulsation.

The first one was a 72 year old diabetic man who had previously suffered two heart attacks and had undergone five coronary artery bypass grafts. His ejection fraction was only 20%. After 35 External CounterPulsation treatments the ejection fraction went up to 36%. While this patient still needs to take a significant number of medications, he is much better off now than he was prior to External CounterPulsation. This also shows that even patients with severe heart disease can usually safely tolerate External CounterPulsation without dangerous side effects.

This second patient was a 27 year old man with angina. Angiograms revealed triple vessel disease with blockages ranging from 95 to 100%. The ejection fraction of this patient was 40%. After 35 External CounterPulsation treatments this patient's angina was completely eliminated at normal levels of activity.

Your grafts are clogging? Don't worry ECP can help.

In 1998 *Clinical Cardiology* published an article demonstrating that patients with triple vessel disease and a prior CABG had a better response to ECP than patients with triple vessel disease without prior CABG. This study suggests that the more blood vessels you have flowing to the heart, the better your response will be to External CounterPulsation even if some of them are partially clogged. Simply stated, this research found that patients with 100% totally blocked arteries responded slower to ECP than patients with coronary blood vessels that were less than 100% blocked. This would suggest that in order for ECP to work effectively some blood flow is necessary. So even if you have had bypass surgery and have had your grafts start to close up again you could still have significant benefit from ECP.

Cut back on your medication.
Doctor Tartaglia from the New York Medical College Department of Cardiology and Doctor Stenerson from the University of Rome published several reports on patients treated with External CounterPulsation. One patient in particular was a 78 year old woman with a history of strokes who had undergone both coronary artery bypass graft and angioplasty. Her angina continued despite the surgeries and she required up to 30 sublingual nitroglycerin tablets per month. Her angina was classified as Canadian Class III which is quite severe. After completing 35 treatments this woman no longer needed any nitroglycerin. The *Journal of Cardiovascular Reviews and Reports* concluded that External CounterPulsation can be a valuable treatment due to the fact that:

- ECP could be done instead of coronary artery bypass grafting and angioplasty

- ECP could also be used to improve the success of CABG and PTCA for those patients that had poor results from the surgery.

Out of an additional 17 patients that were discussed in this review only 2 failed to respond to 35 treatments of ECP and both of these patients had very severe triple vessel disease.

ECP is just as effective as surgery but safer!

The *American Journal of Cardiology* published a study in 1995 which discussed the long term effects of ECP treatment. Patients who had been diagnosed with chronic disabling angina were treated with ECP and then monitored over three years. It was found that the clinical benefits of External CounterPulsation were maintained for at least three years in all patients treated for chronic disabling angina.

Similarly, another study monitored ECP patients for a five-year period and found an 88% survival rate. This finding compares favorably to similar heart patients treated with coronary artery bypass grafting or PTCA where the five-year survival ranged from 86 to 90%.

Researchers at State University of New York (SUNY) at Stonybrook also found out that patients with single or double vessel disease had a success rate of over 90% with 35 External CounterPulsation treatments. Eighty percent of patients with severe triple vessel disease and a history of previous bypass surgery responded to 35 treatments. Only 40% of those with triple vessel disease without previous bypass surgery responded to 35 treatments. This would suggest that patients with severe triple vessel disease probably need 70 or more treatments for the best results.

Want to play tennis?

Many cardiac patients are unable to perform regular daily activities, such as getting dressed, cooking and grocery shopping. These activities are often interrupted by the need to rest because of angina or shortness of breath. The vast majority of patients who are treated with ECP are able to return to normal daily living patterns after they complete their treatments.

Other cardiac patients were once very physical outside of the home. Many participated regularly in sporting events or exercise programs but were forced to discontinue these activities due to cardiac symptoms. Eighty-one percent of patients completing 35 sessions of ECP had an increased ability to exercise. Seventy-eight percent of these patients showed improvement on thallium scanning. It is most likely that had the remaining 19% of the patients continued with additional ECP treatments, the percentage of group improvement could have reached over 90%.

ECP benefits maintained for five years.

In this series of 33 patients treated with ECP by Dr. Lawson and associates 73% had multivessel disease, 45% had prior heart attacks and 61% had either PTCA or CABG. Five years after ECP 64% of the ECP treated patients were found not to have experienced any further major heart events and did not require any additional angioplasty or heart surgery.

Mayo Clinic finds marvelous improvement with ECP.

The Mayo Clinic Division of Cardiovascular Diseases describes the case of a 56-year-old woman who continued to experience severe disabling symptoms of coronary artery disease even though she was taking maximum drug therapy. She needed to take up to four nitroglycerin tablets per day and still experienced angina, even at rest. Aggressive invasive therapies including angioplasty, stents, and quadruple bypass surgery also failed to give this woman relief from her debilitating angina. A nuclear scan of the heart confirmed major circulation defects resulting in insufficient oxygen reaching the heart. Since further surgery was not an option, a course of ECP was prescribed. Following completion of therapy, her angina had declined dramatically and her nuclear scan was normal with complete resolution of the circulation defects. ECP was so effective that this woman is now able to exercise without any limitations. The Mayo physicians concluded that ECP is a safe and effective method for treating angina, even in patients for whom surgery and angioplasty are not suitable.

Johns Hopkins reports remarkable results.

Physicians at Johns Hopkins University Medical School studied the effects of ECP on 18 patients with persistent angina who had previously failed to respond to surgery, angioplasty and maximum medication therapy. Following external counterpulsation, all of the patients showed significant improvement in their cardiac function. As a result, the researchers called for an increase in the availability of ECP therapy across the country.

Thallium scans show improvement after ECP.

Physicians at the Kurume University School of Medicine in Japan performed thallium scans as well as exercise tests on patients both before and after ECP in order to obtain objective evidence of benefit. All the patients studied had significant blockages in major coronary arteries and had been previously treated with medications, angioplasty or bypass surgery. Thirty-five ECP treatments were found to improve exercise tolerance and heart function as well as improved thallium scans.

Depressed? ECP can improve your mood.

It is a well known fact that many patients become severely depressed after a heart attack or after bypass surgery. Doctor Fricchione found that psychosocially, patients did very well with External CounterPulsation. Approximately 67% of External CounterPulsation patients reported an improved social life.

Did someone mention sex?

And researchers from the Department of Urology, Technical University of Dresden, Germany, discovered something interesting while studying ECP and the increased blood flow it provided to the heart. They noticed that ECP also resulted in increased blood flow to the brain, kidneys and penis. Thirteen men with erectile dysfunction received 20 treatments and reported improved erections. Doppler ultrasound confirmed this finding by documenting significant improvement in penile blood flow. The researchers concluded that ECP has the potential to be an effective treatment modality for men with erectile dysfunction.

Congestive heart failure improves with ECP.

John Gorcsan III, M.D., from the University of Pittsburgh, recently presented evidence at the 49th Scientific Session of the American College of Cardiology, which showed that ECP significantly improves congestive heart failure. Patients with congestive heart failure often suffer from fatigue, shortness of breath during normal daily activities, faster than normal heart beat, swelling of the ankles, loss of appetite, and intolerance to cold. Some patients may also wheeze or cough, especially at night after lying down. Heart failure is the most common reason for hospitalization of people over the age of 65.

The patients studied had mild to moderately severe congestive heart failure with an ejection fraction less than forty percent. According to Dr.. Gorcsan, all of the patients treated with ECP showed improvement in the pumping ability of the heart muscle with a corresponding improvement in the ejection fraction. These findings are very exciting because previously the only treatment available for heart failure patients besides drugs and surgery was a heart transplant. Now ECP has been shown to be a safe and effective strategy for improving congestive heart failure. FDA approval is expected soon.

MUST-EECP STUDY.

The *Journal of the American College of Cardiology* published an article in June of 1999, compiling data from The Multicenter Study of enhanced External CounterPulsation (MUST-EECP). Seven prestigious university centers participated in this study:

1. Columbia-Presbyterian Medical Center, Columbia University (New York)
2. Moffit-Long Hospital, University of California at San Francisco (San Francisco)
3. Yale University School of Medicine (New Haven, CT)
4. Beth Israel Deaconess Medical Center, Harvard University (Boston, MA)
5. Grant/Riverside Methodist Hospitals (Columbus, OH)
6. Presbyterian University Hospital, University of Pittsburgh Medical Center (Pittsburgh, PA)
7. Loyola University Medical Center (Maywood, IL).

One hundred-thirty-nine (139) patients with angina, coronary artery disease and positive treadmill tests were selected for this study. The patients were randomly assigned to one of two groups; the first group received actual ECP treatment, and the second group received "sham" or "placebo" treatment. None of the patients knew whether they were receiving legitimate treatment or not.

The results of this study showed that External CounterPulsation effectively decreased angina with many of these patients reporting that the degree of improvement was over 50%. They also reported a decreased need for nitroglycerin and an increased ability to exercise.

Many of the clinical trials validating the efficacy of external counterpulsation therapy since the mid 1990's has been done with equipment supplied by Vasomedical. This includes the MUST-EECP trials, the results of which were published in the *Journal of the American College of Cardiology* in June 1999. Vasomedical continues to lead the way in clinical research on external counterpulsation.

This MUST-EECP study is important because it is the first blinded study to show that External CounterPulsation is effective. This type of study uses two groups of participants, one group receives a placebo (no treatment at all), one group the real treatment; however neither group knows for sure what treatment they are getting. This is what researchers call a "blinded study." A study of this type is unbiased and is usually required by the FDA prior to their approval of any medical device or drug. Yet it is curious that a "blinded study" was never required by the FDA to determine the effectiveness of bypass surgery, angioplasty or stents. In fact, Dr. George E. Burch, from Tulane University School of Medicine, pointed this out in the 1978 issue of the *American Heart Journal*, "There is a definite need for "sham" coronary bypass operations to evaluate coronary bypass surgery." He went on to question why these strict standards of the FDA do not apply to heart surgery. In fact even today some of the drugs used during stent placement surgery are still not FDA approved for that particular use. The bottom line is that with this single blinded study there are now more blinded studies published on ECP than there are for bypass surgery, angioplasty and stents combined!

In an accompanying editorial in the *Journal of the American College of Cardiology*, Dr. C. Richard Conti, a cardiology professor of medicine at the University of Florida Health Science Center, stated, "I believe that enhanced External Counterpulsation has great potential and could be particularly applicable to patients who are not candidates for revascularization but who continue to have repetitive episodes of myocardial ischemia....", "The principle of CounterPulsation has always made great sense to me."

Gregory Barsness M.D., from the Mayo Clinic, one of the most respected medical clinics in the world, has been studying ECP. In an interview in the March 2000 issue of the Rochester Post-Bulletin, Dr. Barsness explains that angina patients have been having dramatic responses to ECP. Out of 21 patients treated with ECP, 20 got better, a success rate of 95%. He goes on to state how the Mayo Clinic is now actively and enthusiastically pursuing ECP therapy for their patients.

Who should decide what treatment you receive?

An article in the *Journal of the American Medical Association* in 1995, stated that treatment of chronic stable angina should be based on the *preferences of the patient*, rather than on the severity of the symptoms alone. These authors from Dartmouth Medical School stated, "the preferences of the individual patient should play a pivotal role in the treatment decision." These doctors should be applauded for this statement. After all, when the health or the life of a patient is at stake, it is the doctor's responsibility to inform the patient of *all* the options, and allow the patient to make the final decision on which treatment they want.

And finally doesn't common sense dictate that one should first try a treatment that is safe, simple, affordable and can be done as an outpatient before trying surgery which is dangerous, costly and often requiring weeks of recovery? In the unusual event that ECP doesn't work then surgery or angioplasty would still be available as a back up plan. ECP is such a safe, effective procedure that it should make surgery and angioplasty a treatment of last resort.

References:

Strobeck JE, Baklajian R, Hannon JC. The emerging role of enhanced external counterpulsation in cardiovascular disease management. The Journal of Cardiovascular Management. 1998;September/October:23-29.

Lawson W, Hui J, Guo T, et al. Prior revascularization increases the effectiveness of enhanced external counterpulsation. Clinical Cardiology 1998;21:841-844.

Strobeck JE, Baklajian R, Hannon JC. The emerging role of enhanced external counterpulsation in cardiovascular disease management. Cardiovascular Reviews and Reports 1997; 1 8(li):20-25.

Tartaglia J, Stenerson JF. Case studies: Enhanced external counterpulsation. Cardiovascular Reviews and Reports 1997;18(11):26-33.

Fricchione GL, Hui JCK, Fife A, et al. Psychosocial aspects of enhanced external counterpulsation. Cardiovascular Reviews and Reports 1997;18(10):37-41.

Lawson WE, Cohn PF, Hui JCK, et al. Enhanced external counterpulsation: U.S. clinical research. Cardiovascular Reviews and Reports 1997; 18(10):25-29.

Cohn PF, Lawson WE, Burger L, et al. Enhanced external counterpulsation: A new therapeutic option for patients who have failed coronary angioplasty and/or bypass surgery. Cardiovascular Reviews and Reports 1997; 18(5):10-17.

Lawson WE, Hui JCK, Oster ZH, et al. Enhanced external counterpulsation as an adjunct to revascularization in unstable angina. Clinical Cardiology 1997;20:178-180.

Lawson WE, Hui JCK, Zheng ZS, et al. Improved exercise tolerance following enhanced external counterpulsation: Cardiac or peripheral effect. Cardiology 1996;87:271-275.

Lawson WE, Hui JCK, Zheng ZS, et al. Three year sustained benefit from enhanced external counterpulsation in chronic angina pectoris. The American Journal of Cardiology 1995;75:840-841.

Conti CAR, Enhanced External CounterPulsation. J Am Coll Cardiol. 1999 Jun;33(7):1841-42.

Arora RR, et al. The Multicenter study of enhanced external counterpulsation (MUST-EECP): effect of ECP on exercise-induced myocardial ischemia and anginal episodes. J Am Coll Cardiol. 1999 Jun;33(7):1833-40.

Froschermaier SE, et al Enhanced external counterpulsation as a new treatment modality for patients with erectile dysfunction. Department of Urology, Technical University Dresden, Germany. Urol Int. 1998;61(3):168-71.

Nease RF Jr, Kneeland T, O'Connor GT, et al. Variation in patient utilities for outcomes of the management of chronic stable angina. Implications for clinical practice guidelines. JAMA 1995 Apr 19;273(15):1185-90

Burch GE. Of the sham operation. Am Heart J. 1978 May;95(5):674.
Singh M, Holmes DR Jr, Tajik AJ, Barsness GW. Noninvasive revascularization by enhanced external counterpulsation: a case study and literature review. Mayo Clin Proc 2000 Sep;75(9):961-5.

Gloth S, Oken HA Enhanced external counter pulsation: the Howard County experience in the first 18 patients. Md Med J 1999 Jul-Aug;48(4):155-6 Johns Hopkins University School of Medicine, USA.

Urano H, Ikeda H, Ueno T, et al. Enhanced external counterpulsation improves exercise tolerance, reduces exercise-induced myocardial ischemia and improves left ventricular diastolic filling in patients with coronary artery disease. J Am Coll Cardiol 2001;37:93-99.

Lawson LE, Hui JCK, Cohn PF. Long term prognosis of patients with angina treated with enhanced external counterpulsation: five year follow-up study. Clin Card 2000;23:254-258.

Chapter 11
Frequently Asked Questions

When did physicians in the United States of America first start treating patients with External CounterPulsation?

The idea of counter pulsation was first thought of in the early 1950's. The Sun Yat-sen University in China was the first to treat patients with ECP in the 1970's and reported over 90% success in patients with angina pectoris.

In 1980 the *American Journal of Cardiology* published a 25-institution multi-center study in which 258 acute heart attack patients were given External CounterPulsation. This was the first major study of its kind in this country. ECP has almost 50 years of research behind it.

Is ECP FDA approved?

Technically the FDA does not approve the actual ECP medical equipment. The FDA does however regulate the marketing and labeling of medical equipment. The FDA first cleared Cardiomedics CardiAssist™ External CounterPulsation device for angina, acute heart attacks and cardiogenic shock in 1987. Vasomedical received clearance in 1995.

How will I benefit?
- Reduction and relief of frequency and severity of angina
- Reduction in chances of dying from a heart attack
- Better treadmill exercise times, able to walk longer and further
- Elimination or reduction of medications used for angina
- Improved blood flow to the heart muscle
- Improvement in quality of life
- Return to former activities like walking, gardening, tennis, golf and swimming
- Some patients also report better vision and improved sexual function

What tests can be done to show that I have improved?

There are several tests that can be done to show improvement after ECP. Your physician could compare before and after ECG's, treadmill tests, thallium or Cardiolite® (technetium-Tc99m sestamibi) scans and perhaps even angiograms. A stress echo could also be used to show improvement.

What is the success rate with ECP?

Studies have shown over 80% of patients have a substantial improvement in their angina symptoms with ECP. This is amazing when one considers that most of these patients had either severe disabling angina or had failed angioplasty or bypass surgery. Just as impressive is the fact that unlike surgery nobody has ever died as a direct result of ECP.

What other conditions besides angina have benefited from ECP?

- Congestive heart failure
- Disabling angina
- Patients with single, double, or triple vessel coronary artery disease
- Patients that respond poorly to medication or do not want to take medication
- Coronary artery heart disease
- Patients who have failed coronary artery bypass graft, stents or angioplasty
- Patients who need to improve their heart circulation prior to surgery
- As an alternative to surgery or angioplasty
- Patients who have failed to respond to chelation therapy
- German studies suggest that ECP may improve erectile dysfunction
- Diabetics often notice faster healing of sores on the feet and improvement of diabetic nerve damage

- Chinese studies suggest that ECP can enhance functioning of the brain, hearing and eyesight as well as lowering high blood pressure.

Experience with athletes suggests that ECP may help speed muscle recovery after prolonged strenuous athletic events such as marathons.

What makes ECP a better treatment for angina than angioplasty, stents or coronary artery bypass grafting?
- No time off work needed - you may do treatments before or after work
- It is an outpatient procedure that has practically no risk
- It is a drug free treatment with no drug side effects
- No surgery or catheters of any kind are required
- Well tolerated by men and women of all ages and body types
- May eliminate or indefinitely postpone the need for bypass surgery or angioplasty.

Is the treatment dangerous? What are the side effects?
When administered properly there are no known significant adverse side effects as a result of treatment with ECP. Patients may however experience minor skin irritation on their legs from the pressure cuff.

Will ECP cause blockages in my blood vessels to break loose?
No, ECP is a very gentle treatment that will not cause any plaque to break free.

How long do the treatments take?
Although the treatments take only one hour, plan on spending at least one and one half-hours in the doctor's office.

What tests do I need before I can start ECP?

You may need most of the following:

- A complete medical history to be taken by the doctor
- Physical exam
- 12 lead ECG
- Blood chemistry including complete blood count, thyroid testing, ferritin and a complete cholesterol profile including HDL, LDL, triglycerides and VLDL
- Additional recommendations may include a treadmill test, echocardiogram, two hour screening for diabetes, testing for homocysteine, Lp(a), apolipoprotein B, LDL pattern testing, etc.
- Abdominal aortic ultrasound may be necessary to check for an aneurysm
- Bilateral venous duplex of the lower extremities to check for possible deep vein thrombosis.

Your doctor will guide you as to the need for these tests.

What do I need to do in order to get ready for a treatment session?

- Arrive 20 minutes early for your appointment
- Continue all your medications. However, your physician may ask you to delay taking your water pills or diuretics until immediately after your treatment
- Don't eat or drink for two hours prior to treatment
- Urinate immediately before getting set up with the pressure cuffs
- Wear easy to change loose clothing, no turtlenecks please. Button-down shirt or blouse is helpful.
- Wear or bring short socks. If you are prone to having cold hands you may also wish to bring mittens
- Men with an excessively hairy chest will need to shave in order to facilitate placement of electrodes for optimal electrocardiogram tracings. The nurse can help you with where you need to shave.

- To prevent chafing your doctor will ask you to apply a water-based lotion the night before and wear tight fitting, full length, stretchy elastic leggings or athletic tights the day of your treatment. If chaffing or irritation becomes a problem then wearing a pair of nylon panty hose under the leggings may be helpful. The ECP nurse will help fit you with the proper size leggings.

What will be done to prepare me for the ECP treatments?
- A therapist obtains your weight and blood pressure
- You change into appropriate clothing and then lie on a padded table
- Two sensors are clipped on your fingers, one to measure blood pressure tracings and another sensor to measure blood oxygen levels. These sensors are painless
- A set of five-blood pressure like cuffs are wrapped around your calves, thighs and buttocks
- Three ECG electrodes are attached to the chest so that your heart rate can be constantly monitored and synchronized with the inflation and deflation of the cuffs on your legs.

The cuffs go through one cycle of inflation and deflation approximately 70 times per minute exactly opposite or counter to your heart rate.

How soon will I start to notice improvements in my angina?
Patients with minimal coronary artery disease often notice improvements after the first fifteen treatments (three weeks). Others with more severe and extensive blockages will often not notice improvements until they have had 35 or more treatments.

How many treatments will I need?
The initial course of treatments is 35 one hour sessions given every day five days a week for seven weeks. Patients with more severe

disease will need to have 70 to 100 one-hour treatments.

Can I skip a few of the 35 treatments to go on a trip?

No. It is very important that you commit to 35 treatments without any interruptions if at all possible.

I'm from out of town; can I do more than one treatment per day?

Although not recommended, some patients are able to take two one-hour treatments per day and can finish in about four weeks. During the first week you will take one treatment per day in order to allow your physician time to assess your response and to let your body adjust to the treatment. If you do well then it may be possible to schedule two treatments a day for the next three weeks. When doing two sessions per day you must have a rest period of 20 minutes between treatments. For most patients it seems that the seven-week treatment protocol works best.

Please note that many insurance companies will not pay for two treatments on the same day.

What does the treatment feel like?

Many people describe the feeling as a deep massage of their legs. It really is similar to the sensation of having your blood pressure taken except that this occurs very quickly in both the calves, thighs and buttocks at the rate of approximately 70 times per minute for one hour. Many patients also experience a flushing of the face.

How will I feel immediately after a one-hour treatment?

After a one hour treatment session you may find that your bladder is full and that you need to urinate. You may also feel somewhat relaxed and fatigued. Occasionally, some patients feel a little light headed immediately after a treatment.

What activities can I do during a treatment session?
- You may listen to music from a compact disk or tape player using earphones
- You may talk to your spouse or friend
- You may go to sleep
- You may wish to listen to a book on tape with headphones.

Will I still need angioplasty or a coronary artery bypass grafting after ECP?
After a successful response to ECP it would be unusual for a patient to require angioplasty or coronary artery bypass graft.

Will I still need to take medications for angina?
Many patients are able to greatly reduce or even eliminate their anti-angina medications after completing ECP.

I've already had coronary artery bypass grafting or angioplasty or stent placement and still have angina and fatigue. Will I still benefit from ECP?
Yes. A study in *Clinical Cardiology* in 1998 showed that ECP was effective in post coronary artery bypass graft patients even when they had extensive coronary artery disease with narrowed grafts. Invasive procedures as mentioned above can only improve blockages in large coronary blood vessels. Small blood vessels with blockages cannot be "fixed" with invasive treatment. ECP however, can provide additional improvement by increasing circulation to areas of the heart not helped with angioplasty, stents or bypass surgery.

My physician says that I must have heart surgery. Will it help to do ECP prior to surgery?
Pretreatment with ECP prior to surgery may be very helpful. Research shows that patients with improved blood supply to the heart do better with surgery and survive heart attacks better with less damage.

Will I need booster treatments after I've completed the prescribed course of therapy?
A three year follow up study published in the *American Journal of Cardiology* showed that clinical benefits of ECP were maintained for almost all patients treated for chronic severe disabling angina. Many patients report benefits continuing for more than five years. It is anticipated however that certain patients may require follow up treatments. A three to seven week session of booster treatments might be necessary for some patients after their initial treatment.

What can I do to maintain the benefits that I have received from ECP and prevent relapse?
- Exercise (walking for instance) to tolerance, six days per week
- Lose weight if needed
- Stress reduction
- Proper diet to optimize your cholesterol HDL, LDL and triglycerides
- Medication if necessary to optimize your cholesterol. Some physicians suggest cholesterol of approximately 150, an HDL greater than 45, an LDL of approximately 80 and triglycerides less than 100
- Aspirin 81 milligrams if tolerated
- Supplementation with vitamin E, coenzyme Q10, magnesium, eicosapentaenoic acid (EPA), niacin, carnitine, hormones, etc. may also be indicated or recommended.

Who is not eligible to have ECP?
Patients with the following may not be suitable candidates for treatment with ECP:
- Aneurysm
- Uncontrolled atrial fibrillation or flutter arrhythmias, frequent premature ventricular contractions

- ECP is not recommended during the first three months immediately following open-heart surgery
- It is also not recommended immediately in the two week period following cardiac catheterization
- Treatment with Coumadin when the INR is greater than 2
- Uncontrolled hypertension or high blood pressure that is greater than 180/110
- Aortic valve weakness or insufficiency
- Pregnancy
- Liver failure
- Phlebitis or deep vein blood clots
- Extremely poor circulation in the legs
- Above the knee amputation of both lower extremities.

I don't want ECP, what are my treatment options?
- Intensive medical treatment with diet, drugs, lifestyle changes and stress reduction
- Angioplasty
- Placement of stents
- Bypass surgery
- Sit back, do nothing, see what happens.

Does insurance pay for ECP treatments?
Many private insurance companies do pay for ECP. Those that won't pay usually do so out of ignorance and unfamiliarity with this new procedure. Efforts to educate them will often result in consideration for payment.

I don't have insurance, can I set up a payment plan?
You may use Visa/Mastercard or one of the following two companies may be contacted for patient financing.

Hillside Patient Financing, 1-800-401-9631
www.affordablepayments.com

Unicorn Financial, 1-888-999-5890
www.howtopayforit.com.

How do I find a doctor that does ECP?
You may contact the two manufacturers of ECP Equipment in the United States.

Cardiomedics Inc.
(provides CardiAssist™ External CounterPulsation)
18872 Bardeen Avenue
Irvine, California 92612
Telephone Number 1-888-849-0200 or 1-949-863-2500
Fax 1-949-474-2274
www.cardiomedics.com

Vasomedical Inc. (Provides EECP®)
180 Linden Avenue
Westbury, New York 11590
Telephone Number 1-800-455-3327 or 1-516-997-4600
Fax 1-516-997-6971
www.eecp.com

How much does a series of 35 treatments cost?
The price varies from office to office but generally ranges from $8,000 to $14,000 per set of 35 treatments. Your condition may require more than one set of treatments. Charges for office visits and lab testing are additional.

I would like to check coverage with my insurance company. What diagnosis codes and common procedural terminology (CPT) codes are used for reimbursement?

International Classification of Diseases (ICD) diagnosis codes that may be used by your doctor are:

- 414.1 Coronary artery disease
- 413.9 Angina pectoris
- 414.9 Ischemic heart disease
- 428.0 Congestive heart failure

CPT codes suggested for External CounterPulsation
Medicare Billing

- G0166   ECP

Commercial Insurance Billing

- 92971   cardioassist method of circulation
- 93922   non invasive volume plethysmography

Does Medicare pay for ECP*? Or what's wrong with this picture?

At this time Medicare will only pay for ECP as a last resort procedure for those patients that are not candidates for surgery or angioplasty and are classified Canadian Angina stage III or IV. Furthermore, a cardiologist must certify that the patient is unresponsive to maximum medical therapy and is not a candidate for PTCA or bypass because the cardiologist believes that:

- the patients condition is inoperable
- there is a high risk of surgical complications
- the anatomy of the blockages is too difficult to bypass
- the patient has other illnesses that make surgery too risky!

*These requirements were in effect at the time this book was written and are subject to change.

It would appear that only the most critically ill heart patients that are beyond the help of a cardiologist or surgeon would be allowed to have ECP! On the one hand this is a tremendous endorsement of the effectiveness of ECP. On the other hand is the fact that under these rules the interventional cardiologist has nothing to lose. It is only those patients on whom the surgeon can no longer perform angioplasty or surgery that Medicare will allow ECP. What this means is that Medicare would rather pay tens of thousands of dollars to the surgeon so that you can first risk your life attempting bypass surgery, angioplasties or stents before consideration is even given to utilizing ECP. Furthermore, once approved by Medicare, only a maximum of 35 ECP treatments are allowed with no additional treatments covered. Doctors familiar with ECP know that severely ill heart patients may need up to seventy or more treatments. What will the consequences be when an ECP physician treats the most critically ill heart patients with the restricted 35 treatments? A patient who might actually need more treatments could fail to improve with such incomplete therapy.

What if similar rules were made to apply to surgeons and interventional cardiologists? What if every potential bypass or stent patient had to get a mandatory second opinion as to the absolute necessity of surgery? What if Medicare told a cardiologist that they were restricted to one stent or one angioplasty with no repeat procedures allowed? Or the heart surgeon being told that even though the patient might benefit from a quadruple bypass Medicare will only allow for one bypass graft per patient and that repeat bypass surgeries are not allowed! How successful do you think bypass surgery would be if these rules were enforced? The truth is that there are no rules like this that apply to surgeons and interventional cardiologists! Only the physicians that do ECP are obligated to follow such a strict set of unrealistic Medicare rules that decides for the physician who they are allowed to treat with ECP and for how long. Who do you want to decide what is best for your health needs, Medicare or your own personal physician?

Moreover, Medicare has strict penalties for doctors that don't follow the rules such as jail sentences and tens of thousand of dollars in fines for each violation! Isn't it ironic that Medicare will gladly pay for multiple angioplasties, stents and three, four or even five repeat bypass surgeries costing tens or hundreds of thousands of dollars. If you survive the first surgery and still have angina, Medicare will allow your physician to prescribe ECP.

Let's just for a moment consider angioplasty, which has a reputation for being less dangerous than bypass surgery. How much more dangerous would it be for a 65-year-old Medicare patient to have angioplasty than a 55-year-old? Well, according to Dr. William S. Weintraub, of Emory University, Atlanta, Georgia, ten-years does make a big difference. The 65-year-old patient has a 65% greater chance of dying after angioplasty than the younger 55-year-old.

The statistics for 80 year-olds undergoing bypass surgery are even worse. Karen P. Alexander, M.D. from Duke University Medical Center, North Carolina, published the following findings in the March 2000 issue of the *Journal of the American College of Cardiology*. Eighty year old patients were found to have a 266% higher chance of dying after a coronary artery bypass graft than younger patients. Complications such as stroke, kidney failure or heart attack occurred twice as often in the 80 year-old patients than it did in the younger patients.

One cardiologist at a meeting was quoted as saying that ECP will be a forgotten treatment in two years. Well, with the interventional cardiologist helping Medicare make the rules restricting access to ECP treatment what else can be expected? The two small companies that make ECP machines and their patients are fighting the medical equivalent of Microsoft®. Unfortunately, this is an example of how politics can affect the practice of medicine.

Not well known among physicians or the public is the fact that the risk of death or heart attack in a person with stable angina or coronary artery disease is only 2% per year. Contrast this with the 4% to 8% risk of death from bypass surgery.

Primum non-nocere -- "first do no harm," is often referred to as the first rule of medicine and has been attributed to Sir William Osler, the father of modern medicine. This Latin phrase states that any treatment or cure should not be worse than the disease being treated. Medicare, by ruling that a patient must first undergo an invasive procedure for heart disease, forces the physician to go against this "first do no harm philosophy." All of us need to do what is best for the patient. Common sense would dictate using a treatment that is safe, simple, and affordable before proceeding to treatments that are dangerous, costly and not always necessary or even beneficial. Why must a patient submit to a dangerous invasive procedure, whether it is bypass surgery, laser, radiation, or angioplasty, when a safer and equally effective alternative therapy is available?

References:
Wientraub WS, et al. Survival after angioplasty drops with increasing age. Am J Cardiol 1999;84:245-251.

Alexander KP, et al. Outcomes of Cardiac Surgery in Patients Age > 80 Years: Results from the National Cardiovascular Network. J Am Coll Cardiol 2000;35:731-738.

Chapter 12

If All You Know is Your Total Cholesterol You Don't Know Enough!

Everyone is usually quite concerned about what his or her total cholesterol levels are. The average person is under the impression that any cholesterol under 200 is acceptable but we will soon find out that it is much more complicated than that. Knowing your total cholesterol is about as useful as knowing the total score of a football game. You have no idea who won or who lost. The same is true with total cholesterol. Someone with a total cholesterol of 165 could still be at a risk for heart attack if the HDL cholesterol is very low. Likewise a total cholesterol of 280 would be probably be nothing to worry about if the HDL is very high, for instance at 100.

HDL cholesterol or high-density lipoprotein is the cholesterol that keeps your arteries clear. Think of the H as standing for "healthy" cholesterol. The HDL cholesterol ratio should be such that when you take your total cholesterol and divide it by your HDL the resultant number should be less than four for a healthy person. Someone who has vascular heart disease should try to obtain a ratio of less than 3. So, in other words, if your cholesterol is 150 your HDL cholesterol should be approximately 50 which gives you a ratio of three. High-density lipoprotein is important because it helps to keep your arteries from clogging. The more HDL you've got, the better. It is worth noting that your total cholesterol and HDL cholesterol can be measured at any time. It is not necessary to fast prior to doing this test. To further complicate this researchers are now finding that there are five different classes of HDL with HDL subclass 2 most often associated with reversal of atherosclerosis.

It is interesting to study primitive societies in third world countries where heart disease and diabetes is almost unheard of. In these societies the total cholesterol rarely exceeds 150. In fact in rural central China the average cholesterol is around 125 and the rate of coronary disease and diabetes is near zero. It is therefore the recommendation of some experts in the field of heart disease prevention that reversal of athrosclerosis is best achieved by a total cholesterol less than 150.

LDL cholesterol, which stands for low-density lipoprotein, is a type of bad cholesterol. One way to remember this is to think of the 'L' standing for 'lousy' cholesterol. It is desirable to have the LDL be below 120 in a person who has never had a heart attack. Research shows that the average heart attack patient has a LDL of 149. However, for people who have cardiovascular disease, had heart surgery, survived a heart attack, or have a family history of heart disease it is recommended by some authorities that the LDL be less than 100. The latest research suggests that even this may be too high and that the LDL should be less than 80.

The most recent research indicates that LDL comes in shades of evil; the smaller the size of the LDL particles the more likely it will cause your blood vessels to clog up. This small dense LDL is called pattern B (think of B for bad). The larger size LDL is less efficient at clogging the blood vessels and is referred to as pattern A (less dangerous than pattern B). One study showed that some patients with pattern A will switch to the more dangerous pattern B when put on a low fat diet. The size of the LDL is determined in part to some extent by your genes and also by your diet. Patients with pattern B often do better on a higher monounsaturated fat diet. Foods emphasized for pattern B patients would be avocados, nuts and seeds, salmon and olive oil.

Lp(a)

Lp(a), called "L, p, little a" is a particularly dangerous form of LDL that enhances blood clotting and contributes to increasing cholesterol deposits in the blood vessel wall. It is noteworthy that niacin, estrogen, testosterone and perhaps coenzyme Q 10 are the only known treatments that will lower Lp(a).

Berkeley Heart Lab in San Mateo, California (800-432-7889) can assist your physician in testing your blood for LDL patterns and HDL subclasses if necessary.

Triglycerides.

Triglycerides are a type of blood fat that many researchers believe to be just as important a risk factor for developing heart disease as cholesterol. It is also a risk factor for developing diabetes. Although opinions vary, many top researchers believe it is desirable for people to have their triglycerides below 100. Unfortunately clinicians in this country do not pay very much attention to triglycerides unless they are exceptionally elevated. Much research shows that triglycerides over 100 with an HDL less than 45 are a significant risk for heart disease. For those people with heart disease reading this book it would be very important to try and achieve triglyceride levels less than 100. The triglyceride/HDL ratio is also important to look at. If triglycerides of 100 are divided by an HDL of 45 the ratio is slightly over 2. It is therefore recommended that an acceptable triglyceride/HDL ratio would be less than 2.5.

It is consequential to note that as the triglycerides go up it causes the HDL to go down. If the triglycerides are over 100 and the HDL is low it will be very difficult to increase the HDL until the triglycerides are reduced! In order to decrease triglycerides, it is often necessary to reduce the consumption of sugar, fruit sugar, fruit juice, and starches (potato, rice, bagels, bread, and pasta) in one's diet. It will also be essential to increase the consumption of certain kinds of "good" fats in the diet. This may come as quite a shock to you that some heart patients might be asked to eat more fat! Research has shown that the Mediterranean people eat a high fat diet yet their rate of heart disease is less than that in the USA. People eating fatty cold water fish also have less heart disease. Not just any fat will do here. The kinds of fats that help improve triglycerides are the monounsaturated omega 9 fats such as olive oil, avocado oil, and the omega 3 cold water fish oil also known as eicosapentaenoic acid (EPA) and docosahexaenoic acid (DHA).

Homocysteine.

One more determinant of cardiovascular risk that needs to be mentioned is homocysteine. Homocysteine is an amino acid (a building block of protein) that is produced in all humans. Some researchers have found that excessively high levels of homocysteine may irritate blood vessels leading to blood clots and blockages in the arteries. It's also known that high homocysteine in the blood can cause cholesterol to change to a form that is more toxic or dangerous to the arteries called oxidized cholesterol. High homocysteine levels may be caused by a dietary lack of B vitamins, especially folic acid, vitamin B6 or vitamin B12. It might also be genetic and may not necessarily be related to diet. Homocysteine is evaluated through a simple blood test that can be measured anytime of the day. It is not necessary to fast prior to doing this test. A healthy homocysteine level is considered to be less than 10 micromoles per liter. A borderline level is 10-12 micromoles per liter of homocysteine. An elevated level of homocysteine would be considered to be over 12 micromoles per liter. If your levels of homocysteine are over 10 it is recommend that you take dosages of folic acid anywhere from 1,000 micrograms (1 milligram) up to perhaps 10,000 micrograms (10 milligrams) or more. Once you have been on your vitamin program for 6-8 weeks it will be necessary for your physician to re-check your homocysteine levels. If the homocysteine levels do not respond to folic acid it may be necessary for your physician to add vitamin B6 (pyridoxine), vitamin B12, or trimethylglycine.

CRP.

C-Reactive Protein is a substance that, when present in the blood serum in abnormal quantities, indicates the presence of inflammation in any of the various body systems. Physicians have used CRP readings for years to assess the degree of inflammation in the joints of patients with arthritis. Now researchers have developed a new version of this simple blood test that measures cardiac CRP or highly sensitive CRP (hs-CRP). Abnormal levels of hs-CRP have been shown to indicate the presence of vascular inflammation and to predict cardiovascular disease and stroke. Just as significant is hs-CRP's role in contributing to these symptoms and conditions. Reducing hs-CRP levels therefore becomes very important since doing so reduces vascular inflammation and one's odds of developing cardiovascular disease or having a stroke. Statin drugs and aspirin can lower hs-CRP levels, and vitamin E may also do so. Dr. Jialal from Texas Southwestern Medical Center found that having patients take 1200 IU of vitamin E daily for three months effectively lowered high levels of hs-CRP.

Syndrome X.
        Another crucial risk factor that is just beginning to get the attention it deserves from physicians is Syndrome X. Dr. Gerald Reaven, professor of medicine and chief of endocrinology at Stanford University, first published an excellent description of this condition in 1988.
        Syndrome X has also been described as the Cardiovascular Dysmetabolic Syndrome, the Insulin Resistance Syndrome or the Deadly Quartet. Syndrome X needs to be taken seriously because it is a very deadly and a very common syndrome affecting as many as one third to one half of the people in this country! Left untreated Syndrome X ultimately leads to **CHAOS**, an acronym that stands for **C**oronary heart disease, **H**ypertension, **A**dult onset diabetes, **O**besity and **S**troke. You do not need to have diabetes or all five of these conditions at the same time to be diagnosed with Syndrome X or insulin resistance. Any one of the above mentioned conditions might indicate that you are insulin resistant and would benefit from

appropriate treatment. Unless this condition is diagnosed and addressed through proper treatment it will be much more difficult to improve your cardiovascular health.

Syndrome X is a metabolic disorder that develops not because a person has too little insulin as happens in juvenile-onset or type I diabetes, but because the body tissues have become resistant to insulin which in turn causes the pancreas to over produce insulin. In some ways it is similar to watering a plant. Too little water and the plant dies, too much water and the plant will also die. This simultaneous resistance to and over production of insulin leads to an accelerated aging process that contributes significantly to the development of heart disease, high blood pressure, stroke and ultimately diabetes.

How do you know if you have Syndrome X?

There are a number of clues that can lead you and your doctor to suspect that you might have Syndrome X. People at risk for Syndrome X are often found to have one or more of the following:

- High triglycerides (over 150)
- Low HDL (less than 45)
- Elevated blood pressure
- Increase in clotting factors, or a tendency to develop blood clots
- Elevated uric acid
- Blood sugars in the fasting state that are over 100 or a two hour glucose tolerance blood sugar over 139
- Fasting insulin levels over 10 or a two hour glucose tolerance insulin level over 30
- Seventy five percent of people with Syndrome X are also overweight
- The following family ancestry, native American Indian, Eskimo, Hispanic, Black, Asian, and northern European especially Finnish, Swedish, Scottish or Irish ancestry
- Family medical histories of diabetes and heart disease
- Women who have had large babies weighing nine pounds or more,

or had pre-eclampsia or toxemia
- Polycystic ovarian syndrome has also recently been associated with insulin resistance.

On physical exam patients at risk for developing Syndrome X are often found to have little tiny projections of skin on their neck or in their armpit area that look like little tiny tags of skin. These skin tags are often a sign of insulin resistance or a diabetic or pre-diabetic condition. Other factors noted on physical exam are a waist/hip ratio in men that is greater than 1 and a waist/hip ratio in women that is greater than 0.8. To put this quite simply, patients at risk for Syndrome X have the shape of an apple rather than the shape of a pear. This means that these patients at risk of Syndrome X carry more of their weight around the abdomen than in their hips and thighs. If you do have Syndrome X aggressive treatment is important because without attention to Syndrome X it will be much more difficult to achieve the optimal levels of cholesterol, triglycerides and HDL needed to reverse your heart disease.

Treatment of Syndrome X or Insulin Resistance Syndrome includes weight loss, exercise, a lower carbohydrate somewhat higher fat diet that uses fats like olive oil and essential fats like cold water fish which supplies eicosapentaenoic acid (EPA). Although not specifically FDA approved for Syndrome X, medications that can be used by your physician to treat insulin resistance include: metformin (Glucophage® Bristol Meyers Squibb), rosiglitazone (Avandia® Smithkline Beecham) and pioglitazone (Actos® Takeda Chemical Industries).

The American Heart Association programs for heart disease prevention.

The following American Heart Association recommendations are presented for comparison purposes because some experts believe that the AHA program does not go far enough in reducing risk factors.

The first program put forth by the AHA is called **Primary Prevention**. This program educates people about risk factors and lifestyle changes to reduce the risk of having a first heart attack. The risk factors that the American Heart Association looks at as contributing to the risk of a person having their first heart attack are as follows:

- Age: for men this would be age 45 years or older, for women 55 years or older
- Hypertension (blood pressure 140/90 mm/Hg or greater although other experts might say 134/84)
- Diabetes (fasting blood sugar over 125, though other experts disagree stating that any fasting blood sugar over 100 is potentially unhealthy. Some authorities think that a two-hour glucose tolerance test is a more sensitive test for diabetes and that any two-hour sugar over 139 should be treated.)
- Smoking
- HDL less than 35 mg per dl (although others suggest less than 45 is unhealthy)
- Family history of coronary heart disease in men under age 50 or women under age 65.

The AHA program for **Secondary Prevention** is involved with identifying and treating patients with established heart disease or those at a very high risk of developing heart disease.

For secondary prevention the American Heart Association recommends:

- LDL less than 100 mg per dl (while other experts suggest that this be less than 80)
- Triglycerides are suggested to be less than 200 mg per dl (other experts suggest that optimal levels are less than 100)
- Physical activity is advocated with a suggested minimum goal of 30 minutes three or four times per week

- Weight management recommendations suggest that patients greater than 125% of ideal weight lose weight.

References:

Miller M, Seidler A, Moalemi A, et al. Normal Triglyceride Levels and Coronary Artery Disease Events: The Baltimore Coronary Observational Long Term Study. J Am Coll Cardiol 1998;31:125-127.

DeFronzo RA, Ferraninini E. Insulin Resistance A Multifaceted Syndrome Responsible for NIDDM, Obesity, Hypertension, Dyslipidemia, and Atherosclerotic Cardiovascular Disease Diabetes Care.1991;14(3):173-194.

Henry RR. Type 2 diabetes care: the role of insulin sensitizing agents and practical implications for cardiovascular disease prevention. Am J Med. 1998;10504 20S-26S.

Reaven GM. Banting Lecture 1988 Role of Insulin Resistance in Human Disease. Diabetes 1988;37:1595-1607.

Bjornholt et al. High-normal blood glucose a risk factor for cardiovascular death Diabetes Care 1999;22:45-49.

Bonora E, Kiechl S, Willeit J, et al. Prevalence of insulin resistance in metabolic disorders: the Bruneck Study. Diabetes 1998 Oct;47(10):1643-1649.

Avignon A, A Radauceanu, L Monnier. Nonfasting Plasma Glucose Is a Better marker of Diabetic Control Than Fasting Plasma Glucose in Type 2 Diabetes. Diabetes Care, December 1997, Volume 20, Number 12, 1822-1826.

High-Dose Vitamin E Reduces Serum Levels of C-Reactive Protein in Diabetes Free Radic Biol Med 2000;8:790-792.

Chapter 13

Natural Therapies that will Further Enhance Your Health and Maintain Your ECP-Derived Benefits

Now that you have achieved improvement in your angina symptoms and have better circulation to the heart it is important that you work at maintaining that improvement. What follows in this chapter is lifestyle, dietary and nutritional suggestions that are crucial to maintaining your new found cardiovascular health.

Exercise.

Probably the single most effective prescription that you can do to die young very old is regular exercise. You plan for retirement by putting money in a 401(k), IRA or some kind of pension plan. Well, what your financial advisor didn't tell you was that at the same time you were making monetary deposits in your pension fund you should also be making exercise "deposits". Regular exercise "deposited" in a 401(h) (401 health plan) or an IHA (Individual Health Account) pays some of the highest yields around. Research has consistently shown that exercise can slow the aging process by an incredible 50%! Thirty minutes of exercise five days per week can decrease your risk for heart attack by 40%. Obviously this is an investment you cannot afford to overlook. The best news is that it is never too late to start.

Under the direction of your physician, start an exercise program as soon as possible. While research has shown that people benefit from 30 minute blocks of exercise new research suggests that smaller units of exercise throughout the day also add up! For instance it is helpful to look for as many excuses as possible to walk an extra few feet.

When going shopping, park your car in the parking space

furthest away. Get rid of the remote control for the TV. When carrying in the groceries from the car, make as many trips as possible. After dinner is over make several trips carrying dishes back to the dishwasher.

Spend more time gardening, take the stairs instead of the elevator, get a dog and take it for a walk; take up square dancing, go for a leisurely stroll, go bowling, golfing, anything to get you on your feet.

It all adds up to make you healthier today and for the future. Just take a few moments to think about the ways you could walk just a little bit further each day. Please start gradually and don't overdo it.

Diet.

Dietary needs vary greatly from one person to another just as does our facial features and shoe size. There is no one diet that will fit everyone. In fact, it has been said that one man's food is another's poison.

Research suggests that there are three major groups of people when it comes to diet. One third of people are in a group that we all seem to hate. These are the people can eat just about anything and not gain weight and still have very good cholesterol numbers. Another one third of people seem to respond extremely well to a very low fat, high carbohydrate, nearly vegetarian diet. The last third of people responds better to a higher fat (good fats like cold water fish and olive oil) and higher protein diet. At first it may be difficult finding the right diet but through careful observation and testing by your physician you should be able to discover the best diet for your personal chemistry. Once you have found a diet that works some customizing or fine-tuning is usually necessary in order to achieve optimal results.

One recommendation that I make to all my patients is that they should eat as many servings of green, yellow and red vegetables per day as possible and to eat less starch, sugar and juice. Many people are surprised by the fact that fruit juice contains more sugar than many soft drinks.

New research is showing that excess consumption of fructose or high fructose corn sweetener found in everything from soft drinks to fruit juice to ketchup to low fat baked goods can raise LDL cholesterol and triglycerides. Many patients lose weight, feel better and have better cholesterol profiles when they greatly decrease the amount of fructose and simple starches consumed. As more research is completed we will see that sugars, simple starches and fructose may be worse for some people than too much fat.

A word about margarine.

You have probably heard that margarine has a type of unsaturated fat called transaturated fat or "trans" fat. Trans fats appear to raise blood cholesterol more than other unsaturated fats and are therefore considered to be just as bad for you as saturated fats. Trans fats are formed when vegetable oil is hardened to become margarine or shortening through a process called hydrogenation. The harder the margarine the more hydrogenated or saturated it is and the more trans fat it has. Please be aware that unlike saturated, monounsaturated or polyunsaturated fats, trans fats are not required to be included on food labels so you have no way of knowing how many grams of trans fats you are consuming. The FDA limits the amount of saturated fat in foods that make a "no cholesterol" or "low cholesterol" claim. But it sets no limit on trans fats. If the FDA counted trans fats along with saturated fat, it would be illegal for many products to be called "no cholesterol" foods. It is best to avoid trans fat and to buy trans fatty acid free spreads that are now readily available in the grocery stores Some examples are Benecol® and Smart Balance®. New legislation will soon force companies to label food with the trans fatty acid content.

Fiber.

There are two types of fiber: insoluble and soluble. Insoluble fiber does not dissolve in water and is found in wheat, corn, rye, rice and many vegetables. Soluble fiber dissolves in water and is found in oat bran, barley, pectin and psyllium. A number of studies show soluble fiber to be very effective and safe in reducing cholesterol and LDL cholesterol. It should be part of any program designed to lower cholesterol. I recommend psyllium to many patients and suggest that they start with one quarter to one half teaspoon per day and very slowly over a few weeks build up to as much as three to six teaspoons or one to two tablespoonfuls per day. Some patients like to take it before meals as it helps fill them up so that they will eat less and lose weight. Other people find it most effective in lowering cholesterol if taken about one hour before bedtime. Psyllium is available as the brand Metamucil® and in many generic forms often labeled natural vegetable powder or fiber.

Soy.

Numerous studies over the past 20 years have shown that soy foods in a diet can lower total LDL cholesterol and increase HDL cholesterol. Soy is a good source of protein and we recommend patients include as much as they can in their diet.

Fish.

There is impressive information supporting substituting fish for beef and pork at least twice a week as a way to reduce heart disease. This benefit first came to light when researchers noticed that Greenland Eskimos on their native high fish, high fat diet had a very low death rate from coronary artery disease. It seems that the omega three fatty acids, eicosapentaenoic acid and docosahexaenoic acid are responsible for this dramatic reduction of heart disease. These two good fats do their job of protecting you from heart attacks by lowering the bloods ability to clot. EPA and DHA in large doses are also very effective at lowering triglycerides. EPA has recently been found to be much more effective than flax oil in reducing triglycerides. Not all fish are equally beneficial. These premium fats are found in fish that live in cold water. The best fish for omega three oils are salmon, halibut, cold lake trout, sardines, mackerel and herring. For patients that have a severe triglyceride problem I will often recommend 1,500 to 3,000 milligrams of EPA per day. Please read the label on your supplement carefully. While many bottles state that each capsule of fish oil contains 1000 milligrams of omega three usually only 180 to 360 milligrams of that is the beneficial EPA. One side effect of too much EPA is diarrhea which requires using a smaller dose. The problem some people experience with fish oil, burping or belching, can usually be solved by taking the capsules frozen with food or prior to going to bed at night. Note: Since omega three oils are very unsaturated it is very important to supplement your diet with at least 400 international units of vitamin E in order to keep the oils from becoming rancid in your body.

Saturated fat.

Replacing saturated animal fat in a diet with large quantities of fat free carbohydrates has been shown to reduce the levels of the healthy cholesterol, HDL. Patients will often notice an increase in their HDL when replacing animal fats with olive or canola oil and eating more cold water fish. If you find that the HDL is going down on your present diet talk to your doctor about including some additional good oils and see if your HDL rises.

Vitamin E.

Vitamin E is probably the single most important vitamin for anyone with cardiovascular disease to take. It is a powerful antioxidant and is thought to decrease heart attacks by preventing LDL cholesterol from oxidizing. Much research has shown that oxidized LDL cholesterol is more dangerous than non-oxidized LDL. Think of rusted iron as representing oxidized LDL. Now think of iron with a nice clean coat of paint protecting it from rusting. This is similar to what vitamin E does for LDL cholesterol, it keeps it from rusting or oxidizing.

Two studies published in the *New England Journal of Medicine* look at the relationship between vitamin E and heart disease in 87,000 female nurses and 39,000 male health care professionals. These studies showed that up to a 40% reduction in coronary disease was noted in those people taking more than 100 international units of vitamin E per day. The Cambridge Heart Antioxidant Study revealed a significant reduction in non-fatal heart attacks when patients with known heart disease were taking 400 to 800 international units of vitamin E per day. Although the research is not completely clear as to what type of vitamin E is best I've been recommending natural d-alpha tocopherol with mixed tocopherols.

Niacin, Vitamin B3.

While niacin is probably one of the most effective natural substances for reducing LDL, triglycerides and Lp(a) it is also probably one of the most potentially hazardous natural substances. Large doses of niacin can cause gastrointestinal upset, nausea, elevated blood sugar, gout and occasionally vitamin induced hepatitis in susceptible people.

Since large doses of niacin are required to have the desired effect on your cholesterol it is best that you take large doses of this vitamin under the care of a physician. One unique effect of large doses of niacin in most people is that it causes a rather harmless yet annoying hot, flushing, itching, tingling sensation that lasts for about 30 minutes before disappearing. This niacin flush can often be prevented by one of the following: take aspirin 30 to 60 minutes prior to taking the niacin or take inositol hexanicotinate, a form of niacin that does not cause flushing. Another option is the newly FDA approved time release niacin, Niaspan® by Kos Pharmaceuticals. Taking niacin in a time release form can reduce the severity of flushing. The optimal time to take Niaspan® is at bedtime or after a snack. Therapy with Niaspan® is best initiated by having your doctor prescribe the starter pack in order to reduce the incidence of flushing.

Although niacinamide is also a form of vitamin B3 do not substitute it for niacin since it will have no effect whatsoever on your cholesterol.

Pyridoxine (Vitamin B6), Folic acid, Vitamin B12.
All the B complex vitamins such as Thiamine (B1), Riboflavin (B2), Niacin (B3), Pyridoxine (B6), Cobalamin (B12), Folic Acid, Biotin and Pantothenic acid are important. However folic acid, vitamin B12 and vitamin B6 are the most important vitamins for lowering levels of homocysteine. Found in everyone's blood, homocysteine damages blood vessels when levels exceed 10. Homocysteine is thought to cause problems by contributing to atherosclerosis and blood clots. While homocysteine levels can usually be normalized with small doses of folic acid some patients with exceedingly high levels of homocysteine need 1,000 to 25,000 micrograms (1 to 25 milligrams) per day of folic acid in order to bring their homocysteine levels down to less than 10.

Vitamin C.
This is an interesting vitamin because all animals except man, primates, guinea pigs, fruit eating bats and salmon can make their own vitamin C. Apparently somewhere along the way our liver lost the ability to make vitamin C. Vitamin C like vitamin E acts as an antioxidant, however vitamin C is a water soluble antioxidant unlike vitamin E which is fat soluble. Vitamin C can help lower LDL cholesterol and also seems to protect the inside lining of the many miles of blood vessels in our bodies. Many physicians recommend 1,000 to 3,000 milligrams per day.

Coenzyme Q10.
Coenzyme Q10 is a potent antioxidant that is made by every cell in our bodies. As we age the levels of this antioxidant decreases. People taking statin drugs to lower cholesterol should be aware that

statins, while decreasing production of cholesterol in the liver also decreased the production of CoQ10. For this reason, I recommend that all patients on cholesterol lowering drugs take about 100 milligrams of CoQ10 to compensate for any decreased production of this vital substance.

CoQ10 has been shown to improve the function of weak heart muscles such as occurs in heart failure, reduce episodes of angina, and improves survival in patients after heart attacks. CoQ10 may also be useful in unhealthy levels of Lp(a). Other research suggested it might also be helpful in cancer patients.

L-Carnitine.

L-Carnitine is a protein-like substance that transports fat into the mitochondria where energy is produced. Heart patients given 2,000 milligrams of carnitine per day are able to exercise longer with less angina. L-carnitine can also lower LDL cholesterol, triglycerides, and raise HDL. It is exceptionally safe and is available over the counter.

Arginine.

Patients with severe Stage III and Stage IV angina have been shown to improve dramatically with the use of up to 9 gm arginine per day. In large doses arginine has been found to prevent blood clotting and improves blood flow by increasing nitric oxide. This natural amino acid seems to be well tolerated and even at this high dose almost no side effects were noted. Arginine powder is available in many health food stores. Because arginine is found in fish and meat some vegetarians may be deficient in this amino acid.

Magnesium.

Magnesium is probably one of the most important minerals for any heart patient. Even the slightest deficiency can cause problems. Numerous studies have shown that magnesium is valuable in treating palpitations, arrhythmias, angina, chest pain, mitral valve prolapse, hypertension and blood vessel spasms. It is a critical mineral for patients with diabetes.

Blood tests and most other tests are not very accurate ways to diagnose magnesium deficiency since only 1% of the body's total magnesium is in the blood or serum. Ninety-nine percent of the body's magnesium is in the muscles, brain and bone. In other words, your blood test could show that your magnesium levels are fine when in fact they are low.

Suggested amounts for most healthy people is about 300 mg of elemental magnesium per day. If you are ill you may require much more than that. People with kidney failure require less. Too much oral magnesium can cause diarrhea that may eventually lead to a deficiency of magnesium. Do not take magnesium supplements if your kidneys do not function properly.

Calcium.

Calcium, like magnesium is also important for the heart. Research has shown that calcium supplements can help to lower blood pressure, prevent colon cancer, prevent osteoporosis and help to lower blood cholesterol by binding cholesterol containing bile salts in the intestines. Suggested dosages range from 800-2,000 mg per day.

Potassium.

Potassium is another critical mineral and works best in tandem with magnesium. Potassium has been shown to reduce blood pressure, prevent strokes, and relieve muscle cramps and weakness. Many diuretics tend to deplete the body of potassium and magnesium. It is often necessary that patients taking water pills or diuretics supplement with extra potassium and magnesium. Vegetable foods are a good source of potassium. Too much potassium can be dangerous so please check with your physician before taking large quantities of this mineral.

Chromium.

Chromium is helpful to the heart patient in a number of ways. Many studies have shown that chromium can raise HDL cholesterol, lower LDL cholesterol and triglycerides as well as improve blood sugar and insulin sensitivity in diabetics. Dosage ranges from 200 to 600 mcg.

Selenium.

Selenium and vitamin E work very closely together as powerful antioxidants and for that reason only it would be very important for heart patients to take. By preventing oxidation of LDL cholesterol the risk of arterial damage decreases. Other research has shown that selenium can decrease the risk of prostate cancer. Supplemental dosages of this mineral are very small, usually less than 200 micrograms per day.

Natural Statins.

Chapter 14 discusses statins, a very powerful class of medications used by physicians to lower cholesterol. Cholestin® is a natural alternative to prescription statins marketed by Pharmanex, Inc. This natural statin is a product of rice fermentation and can be used to reduce elevated cholesterol levels of 200-240 mg/dl. Studies show that this supplement can reduce overall cholesterol by 15 to 30 percent and LDL by 22 percent. Cholestin® is less costly than its prescription alternative and therefore may be a cost-saving option for some patients. Although no serious side effects have been noted in Cholestin® users, it may prudent for your physician to monitor liver and muscle enzymes while you take it.

There are many suggestions in this chapter and you may be eager to begin them all at once. Please be patient and begin gradually when starting exercise, making diet changes and adding supplements. Please be sure to check with your physician before beginning anything recommended in this book.

References:
Rimm EB, Stampfer MJ, Ascherio A, et al. Vitamin E consumption and the risk of coronary heart disease in men. N Eng J Med 1993;328:145-146.

Stephens NG, Parsons A, Schofield PM, et al. Randomised controlled trial of vitamin E in patients with coronary disease: Cambridge Heart Antioxidant Study (CHAOS) Lancet 1996 Mar 23;347(9004):7816.

Stampfer MJ, Hennekens CH, Manson JE, et al. Vitamin E consumption and the risk of coronary disease in women. N Engl J Med 1993;328:144-149.

Mortensen SA, Leth A, Agner E, Rohde M. Dose-related decrease of serum coenzyme Q10 during treatment with HMG-CoA reductase inhibitors. Mol Aspects Med 1997;18 Suppl:S137-44.

Heber D, et al. Cholesterol-lowering effects of a propriety Chinese red-yeast-rice dietary supplement. Am J Clin Nutr 19999;69:231-6

Chapter 14
The Amazing New Cholesterol Lowering Medications

Sometimes, despite everything we try the blood cholesterol levels still cannot be optimized. This is where new, powerful and effective medications can be prescribed. Many of you reading this book may be reluctant to take medications, but for heart patients the benefits of these new medications usually far out weigh any side effects. If you are to achieve your goal of a heart healthy future then please give serious consideration to a comprehensive program that just may have to include some pharmaceuticals. In fact, the research on the effectiveness of drugs in preventing heart attacks is so convincing it would be unthinkable not to suggest them to a patient at high risk of having a heart attack or stroke.

How low should cholesterol be?

To review what optimal levels for lipids should be let's listen to what William T. Castelli, M.D., internationally recognized researcher, medical director of the Framingham Cardiovascular Institute, associate professor of medicine Boston University and a regular lecturer at Harvard Medical School for over 35 years, has to tell us. Dr. Castelli recommends that heart patients have the following goals:

- Total cholesterol of 150 or less
- Ratio of total cholesterol to HDL less than 3 (total cholesterol divided by HDL)
- LDL at 100 or less
- Triglycerides 100 or less.

Dr. Castelli is not alone in these recommendations. K. Lance Gould, M.D. from the University of Texas Medical School has even stricter criteria. Dr. Gould, in an article published in the *American*

Journal of Medicine explains that coronary artery disease can be successfully treated without surgery if the following parameters, which are based on an extensive review of the literature and his own personal experience, are attained:

- Lose weight if needed in order to achieve a lean body weight
- Total cholesterol should be less than or equal to 140
- LDL less than 90
- HDL greater than 45.

A patient achieving these numbers through aggressive medical treatment has a greater than 90% probability of partial regression of coronary artery disease or at the very least no progression along with no more heart attacks or angina. For those readers that would criticize this as being too aggressive let me remind them that this is still much less aggressive, less dangerous, less expensive and more effective in the majority of heart patients than either angioplasty or bypass surgery! Dr. Gould goes on to state, "...this treatment paradigm might be called a 'reversal treatment' for coronary atherosclerosis in that it markedly decreases symptoms and the probability of MI, death, PTCA, or CABG, and is a relatively low-cost alternative to traditional invasive approaches." He further argues that, "...the current, primarily invasive approach based on coronary arteriography and revascularization procedures is outmoded and inadequate in the face of new clinical algorithms utilizing vigorous lipid and risk factor control as an alternative to invasive procedures for the primary treatment of CAD."

Patients with very elevated cholesterol usually need medications to achieve optimal lipid levels. And for heart patients the latest research shows that the benefits of these medications far outweigh any risks or side effects. Please remember that treatment with these medications will most likely be life long. Should you decide for whatever reason to stop cholesterol-lowering medications then your cholesterol will return to its previously elevated level and greatly increase your risk for a heart attack.

Statins

Statins, also known as HMG CoA reductase inhibitors are very powerful medications when it comes to treating cholesterol problems. The following is a list of the currently available statins.

- Atorvastatin, brand name Lipitor™ Parke Davis, supplied as tablets of 10mg, 20mg, 40mg
- Cerivastatin, brand name Baycol™ Bayer Corporation, supplied as tablets of 0.2mg, 0.3mg, 0.4mg
- Fluvastatin, brand name Lescol® Novartis Pharmaceuticals, supplied as capsules of 20mg, 40mg
- Lovastatin, brand name Mevacor® Merck and Co., supplied as tablets of 10mg, 20mg, 40mg
- Pravastatin, brand name Pravachol® Bristol Myers Squibb, supplied as tablets of 10mg, 20mg, 40mg
- Simvastatin, brand name Zocor® Merck and Co., supplied as tablets of 5mg, 10mg, 20mg, 40mg.

Statins are the most effective drugs available for lowering LDL and total cholesterol. In the last few years many studies have been published showing the effectiveness of these medicines in preventing heart attacks and reducing the risk of stroke. The results of utilizing statins are very impressive. Appropriate use of statins in numerous studies has been shown to:

- Reduce the risk of coronary heart death by up to 45%
- Reduce risk of stroke by as much as 40%
- Decrease risk of heart attack by over 40%
- And reduce the need for angioplasty and bypass surgery by as much as 37%.

Other studies have clearly illustrated that for every 1% decrease in cholesterol there is a 2% decrease for coronary heart disease. For example, a decrease in cholesterol by 25% would decrease the risk of heart attack by 50%.

Although every drug, vitamin, herb or mineral is capable of producing side effects many statin users experience little or no side effects. The frequency and severity of side effects depends on dose, length of therapy and individual susceptibility. You should notify your physician immediately if any of the following happen: muscle pain, muscle weakness, nausea, vomiting, fevers or unexplained headaches. Since these medications may cause sun sensitivity use sun screens and avoid prolonged exposure to the sun. At one time it was also thought that very low levels of cholesterol were associated with excess cancer deaths and excess trauma deaths. However, the latest research shows no connection between cholesterol lowering drugs and excess non-cardiovascular deaths or psychological problems.

It will be necessary for your physician to periodically monitor liver and perhaps muscle enzymes while on these medications.

The value of getting cholesterol levels to 150 mg or lower in preventing or arresting coronary heart disease is illustrated quite nicely in this study from the Cleveland Clinic. Eleven patients with severe triple vessel coronary artery disease were treated with medication in order to achieve cholesterol levels of less than 150. In the years prior to this study these 11 patients with an average age of 56 years had an amazing total of:

- 8 cases of bypass surgery
- 2 cases of angioplasty
- 15 periods of worsening angina
- 4 heart attacks
- 3 strokes.

For 10 years these patients were treated with diet and medications in order to maintain cholesterol of less than 150. The 6 patients that stuck with the program had absolutely no further heart problems at all during this ten year period. However, the 5-drop out patients reported:

- 4 episodes of worsening angina
- one bypass
- one angioplasty
- one heart failure

- one death from heart rhythm problems
- and 2 episodes of heart rhythm irregularities.

Fibrates

There are presently two fibrates available in this country. Fenofibrate or Tricor™ (Abbott Laboratories) and gemfibrozil or Lopid® (Parke-Davis). Both of these medications are useful when a person has high triglycerides that do not respond to diet, statins or fish oils. A recent study of over 2,500 men showed that gemfibrozil decreased deaths from heart attacks and strokes by 24%. While earlier studies showed that there might be an increased risk of cancer, this study showed that the gemfibrozil group actually had a slightly lower incidence of cancer.

The Helsinki Heart Study showed a 71% reduction in heart attacks when gemfibrozil was used. Gemfibrozil and fenofibrate are particularly useful in patients with Syndrome X also known as Insulin Resistance Syndrome.

Other medications that can be useful.

Orlistat® (Roche) or Xenical is a FDA-approved medication for weight loss. This medication works by preventing an intestinal enzyme called lipase from breaking down fat so it can be absorbed. If you are unable to absorb the fat in your intestines then fewer calories will be absorbed and you may lose some weight. Some side effects of this medication include oily spotting, fatty or oily stool and more frequent bowel movements. In addition to facilitating weight loss this medication has also been shown to improve lipid profiles in patients and improve blood sugar control in diabetics.

Robert R. Henry, M.D., believes that there is a real advantage in treating the insulin resistance component of cardiovascular disease with an insulin sensitizer like Glucophage® or Metformin or maybe even one of the "glitazones". Typically used in type II diabetics, Dr. Henry suggests that these medications may be very useful in coronary heart patients with insulin resistance because it can significantly improve the lipid profile. As a side benefit many patients taking metformin find it much easier to lose weight. Although only FDA approved for diabetes, many physicians have found insulin sensitizers helpful in treating patients with coronary artery disease.

Aspirin

Blood clots are one of the major contributors to a sudden heart attack. Aspirin blocks an enzyme in platelets that keeps them from clumping and forming a blood clot. Research has shown that a daily dose of 81 milligrams of aspirin will do the trick in preventing or reducing the development of blood clots. For an acute heart attack chew a 325 milligram aspirin tablet, after dialing 911, while waiting for the ambulance. Aspirin is also helpful in preventing strokes that are caused by blood clots and may prevent colon cancer. Please do not substitute Tylenol or acetaminophen since it has no effect on blood clotting.

Conclusion

Whatever you and your physician decide to do, it is important to remember that once your cholesterol is at goal and you feel better, that is not the time to quit. Your diet, exercise program, nutritional supplements and medications will most likely be an ongoing treatment for the rest of your life. And remember, follow up with your physician on a regular basis even if you feel well.

References:
Esselstyn CB Jr, Ellis SG, Medendorp SV, Crowe TD. A strategy to arrest and reverse coronary artery disease: a 5-year longitudinal study of a single physician's practice. J Fam Pract 1995 Dec;41(6):560-568.

Rubins HB. et al. Gemfibrozil reduces risk of coronary events in men with CHD and low HDL levels. N Engl J Med 1999;341:410-418.

Gould LK. New concepts and paradigms in cardiovascular medicine: the noninvasive management of coronary artery disease. Am J Med 1998;104(6A): 2-17

Henry RR. Type 2 Diabetes Care: The Role of Insulin Sensitizing Agents and Practical Implications for Cardiovascular Disease Prevention. Am J Med. 1998;10504 20S-26S.

Chapter 15

Sex Hormones: Not Just for Sex and No Longer the Heart's Enemy

Natural Testosterone and Male Cardiovascular Disease

The medical establishment has assumed for years that testosterone plays a major role in worsening cholesterol levels and causing coronary artery disease and heart attacks in men. In fact, just the opposite may be true. New research is showing that low testosterone may actually increase a man's risk of developing coronary atherosclerosis. This makes basic sense when one considers that the heart is a muscle and that testosterone enhances muscular growth and performance.

The Research

In a study published in the June 2000 issue of the *European Heart Journal*, researchers compared the testosterone levels of 30 healthy men and 60 men with proven coronary artery disease. Testosterone levels were found to be significantly lower in the men with heart disease, corroborating the findings of a 1996 Polish study and a 1998 Chinese study, both of which concluded that low testosterone is a risk factor for coronary artery disease. In another study conducted by some of the same researchers and published in the October 2000 issue of *Circulation*, the relationship between low testosterone and cardiovascular disease was found to be even more significant. In this study men with chronic stable angina were given either low-dose transdermal testosterone therapy or a placebo and asked to answer quality-of-life questionnaires regularly throughout the experience. The men given real testosterone patches showed a substantial increase in their ability to exercise, reported less angina, and scored considerably higher on the quality-of-life questionnaires than the men given the placebo. In addition, there were no detrimental changes noted in blood counts or lipids. The researchers concluded that significant numbers of men with cardiovascular disease might benefit from testosterone replacement therapy. Those who stand to gain the most, in fact, may be those with the lowest testosterone levels, according to a 1999 Italian study also published in *Circulation.*

Other Potential Roles for Natural Testosterone in Heart Treatment.

Natural testosterone is showing itself to be useful in the treatment of a variety of heart ailments and may one day be considered a cardiovascular drug, according to researchers at the Albert Einstein College of Medicine. A review of the scientific literature on the subject by these physicians found that so-called healthy men with low testosterone had higher blood sugars, elevated triglycerides, higher total cholesterol and LDL cholesterol. On the other hand, it was found that the administration of testosterone to raise levels to a mid-normal range decreased total cholesterol and LDL, increased HDL cholesterol, and augmented the fibrinolytic system which helps prevent clots. The previously mentioned Polish study also found that testosterone replacement therapy decreased total cholesterol and LDL while not having any adverse effects on HDL. The University of California, San Diego also reviewed the published data on testosterone and found that testosterone either had no effect or a beneficial effect on HDL levels. The reviewers also found that testosterone would help relieve angina and, in addition, associated higher testosterone levels with lower systolic blood pressure.

Other research found that men with congestive heart failure might also benefit from taking testosterone due to the beneficial effect it has on both the skeletal system and the cardiac muscle. A separate study published in the May 2000 *American Geriatric Society Journal* discovered that men over 65 undergoing cardiac rehabilitation responded better to the program and had more muscle strength when they were given supplemental testosterone.

Abnormal electrical heart patterns may also be regulated by supplemental testosterone, according to a report in the October 2000 issue of the *American Heart Journal*. In this report ECG patterns were also shown for the first time to be abnormal in men with low levels of testosterone. It appears testosterone may have yet another role in the treatment of heart conditions.

Testosterone Testing.

Testosterone levels can be easily measured through blood or saliva testing. However when ordering blood testing, it is important for your physician to specify that the lab test for "free testosterone" as opposed to total testosterone since free testosterone represents the bioavailable or active hormone, that is, the testosterone available or not available to help your heart function properly. Salivary analysis for testosterone is proving to be a very practical, easy and affordable way to check levels. Care needs to be exercised when evaluating testosterone levels because men do not experience the rapid, sudden onset of the change of life that women do. Instead there is a progressive decline in testosterone levels over a thirty- to forty-year period. This makes it much more difficult to ascertain exactly when a man's testosterone becomes too low.

Men taking natural testosterone should also have their PSA or prostate specific antigen monitored regularly along with their blood count. It is possible that administering testosterone could increase the risk of prostate cancer or prostate enlargement, cause an elevated blood count, or decrease sperm count. Regular blood testing would allow for early detection and treatment of these occasional reactions to testosterone therapy.

A final comment: anyone contemplating testosterone replacement therapy should in no way confuse it with the abuse of synthetic anabolic steroids such as that which occurs in the sports arena. The latter abuses and overdoses on synthetic testosterone; the former uses natural testosterone in normal doses.

Women, Estrogen and Cardiovascular Disease.

Although a clear cause and effect relationship is not yet proven, strong evidence exists that hormone replacement therapy lowers the risk of coronary heart disease in women without a personal history of heart disease. In fact estrogen is one of the few treatments that can be used to normalize elevated levels of Lp(a) thereby reducing the risk of coronary artery disease. Remember that more women die from heart disease than from all forms of cancer put together. Instead of studying women with no heart disease, the Heart and Estrogen/progestin Replacement Study (HERS) looked at women that had established heart disease. These women took horse estrogen and synthetic medroxyprogesterone and were found to have a greater risk of heart disease—but only in the first four months. At the end of four years, however, there was a trend toward decreasing risk. More studies are needed to further evaluate this intriguing effect.

It is important to note that female hormone replacement therapy may raise the risk of venous blood clots although this risk is exceedingly small in healthy women. Also, taking a baby aspirin (81 mg), vitamin E and eating cold water fish such as salmon twice a week or taking fish oil supplements could help prevent such clotting.

References:
Lancet 1999: 354: 152-55. Clinical Synthesis Panel on Hormone replacement Therapy Division of Epidemiology & Biostatistics, European Institute of Oncology, Milan Italy

English KM, Mandour O, Steeds RP, Diver MJ, Jones TH, Channer KS. Men with coronary artery disease have lower levels of androgens than men with normal coronary angiograms. Eur Heart J 2000 Jun;21(11):890-4

English KM, Steeds RP, Jones TH, Diver MJ, Channer KS. Low-dose transdermal testosterone therapy improves angina threshold in men with chronic stable angina : A randomized, double-blind, placebo-controlled study. Department of Cardiology, Royal Hallamshire Hospital, Sheffield, UK (K.M.E., R.P.S., K.S.C.).Circulation 2000 Oct 17;102(16):1906-11

Rosano GMC, Leonardo F, Pagnotta P, Pelliccia F, Panina G, Cerquetani E, et al. Acute anti-ischemic effect of testosterone in men with coronary artery disease. Circulation 1999;99:1666-70.

Bakhshi V, Elliott M, Gentili A, Godschalk M, Mulligan TJ. Testosterone improves rehabilitation outcomes in ill older men. Am Geriatr Soc 2000 May;48(5):550-3

Shapiro J , Christiana J , Frishman WH. Testosterone and other anabolic steroids as cardiovascular drugs. Department of Medicine, the Albert Einstein College of Medicine, Bronx, New York, USA. Am J Ther 1999 May;6(3):167-74

Zgliczynski S, Ossowski M, Slowinska-Srzednicka J, Brzezinska A, Zgliczynski W, Soszynski P, Chotkowska E, Srzednicki M, Sadowski Z. Effect of testosterone replacement therapy on lipids and lipoproteins in hypogonadal and elderly men. Atherosclerosis 1996 Mar;121(1):35-43

Barrett-Connor EL. Testosterone and risk factors for cardiovascular disease in men. Department of Family and Preventive Medicine, University of California, San Diego Diabete Metab 1995 Jun;21(3):156-61.

Chapter 16

Guide to Insurance Reimbursement for ECP

Most insurance is usually a contract between the patient and their insurance company. (This is in contrast to HMO's where the physician, also called a gatekeeper, is part of the contract and is usually encouraged to limit care in order to keep costs down.) With private insurance the physician is not part of that contract, it is your insurance not the doctors. And while it is helpful for your physician to write a letter to your insurance company it is much more effective if you, the policyholder or the person that pays the premiums, write a letter directly to the insurance company.

Before writing to the insurance company please take time to study your plan's benefits booklet. Patients often assume that just because a physician prescribes a treatment or medication it will automatically be covered. However, if your insurance contract specifically states that a certain procedure or medication is strictly excluded then having your physician write a letter or filing a complaint will not help. Procedures or medications that are not covered or are only partially covered become the financial responsibility of the patient.

Even if the insurance covers the procedure there are still co-pays and deductibles that affect your out of pocket expenses. Generally more expensive policies have expanded benefits and lower co-pays. In other words, you get what you pay for. Therefore, it is very important that you obtain a copy of your insurance benefits and read them carefully. Does your benefit plan have language such that ECP might be considered for payment? Knowing what is stated in your explanation of benefits can be very useful information when writing your insurance company a letter. The following approach has helped many patients obtain coverage for ECP.

When corresponding with the insurance company be sure to include:

- Your name, address and phone number
- Social security number
- Date of birth
- Group or subscriber number
- Policy number, name and type of policy.

For all phone conversations keep written notes of:
1. The date and time of your call
2. The phone number called with extension
3. Name, department and job title of the person you talked to
4. Details of what was discussed and what action was going to be taken
5. Keep copies of everything.

Send copies of any letters to your employer's benefits manager or human resources director. The benefits manager may have some leverage with the health plan, since employers can consider switching health plans if there are enough complaints.

In your initial request for coverage write the insurance company a letter stating the following:

- Explain how your heart condition affects or limits your daily life physically, socially and mentally
- List the number of medications you need to take for your condition
- Explain that your physician believes that this treatment is medically necessary
- Describe how ECP is much less expensive than a $20,000 angioplasty or a $70,000 bypass surgery and that ECP is much safer
- List the following CPT codes that you are requesting coverage for:
  92971 Cardioassit method of circulation
  93040 ECG

93922 Plethysmography
94761 Pulse oximetry
99211 -25 E/M RN
99215 -25 E/M Physician

- Explain that the procedure is FDA "cleared to market" and is a covered benefit of Medicare
- Politely request that your insurance company pay for your treatment
- Include information from your physicians about your condition
- If you have already completed treatment explain how it has helped you.

In most states health insurance plans have a limited time (usually 2 to 14 days) in which to respond and must notify you of their decision in writing or by fax. Make sure any denial of your initial request includes:

- The main reason(s) for the refusal to pay for the treatment
- How to initiate your first appeal
- How to obtain a written statement of the clinical criteria used in the decision
- Who made the decision to deny your claim and their qualifications. If it was a committee that made the decision find out who the members were and their training. Are they at all familiar with ECP?

When filing your first appeal ask that your appeal be evaluated by a physician who was not involved in the first decision to deny your claim. If the first appeal is denied make sure you have the following information:

- Name title and qualifications of the doctor who evaluated the appeal
- The reviewer's statement of the reason for the appeal
- The medical reason for the decision
- How to file a second level appeal.

If you are still not satisfied then you may or may not be able to file a second level appeal depending upon the insurance rules in your state. Please note that under federal law known as ERISA state insurance laws do not apply to self-insured health plans. Many large insurance corporations offer plans that are self-insured. To find out if your company is self-insured contact your employer's human resources department. These plans have their own appeals procedures. Second level appeals vary from state to state. Some plans must appoint a grievance review panel of three or more health professionals with the appropriate expertise that were not involved in the original denial, are not employees of the health plan and do not have a financial interest in the outcome. The panel must meet within a specified number of days and you usually have the right to appear in person before the panel. You may or may not be able to have your attorney present.

If you are still dissatisfied then you may wish to contact your State Division of Insurance. The division of insurance can:
- Record your complaint against the health plan
- Investigate your complaint
- Make sure that you get clear answers to your questions
- Make sure that state law is followed.

The division of insurance cannot:
- Force a favorable decision if the law and the facts are not on your side
- Require your plan to pay for services that are excluded by your policy
- Provide legal services.

Do not give up after the first denial. Keep writing and calling since you have nothing to lose. Persistence can pay off.

Appendix
Physicians, Universities and Hospitals That Provide External CounterPulsation

Since you can't readily find a physician that uses ECP in the yellow pages I've provided the following addresses and phone numbers. Please contact the companies directly for a listing of physicians in your geographic area that performs ECP.

Note: Recommendation of a physician by the manufacturer does not signify the author or publisher's endorsement of a particular physician's expertise or competence. Likewise, being listed here does not signify that the companies or the physicians or clinics that are recommended endorse or authorize any or all of the material presented in this book.

You may contact the following manufacturers of ECP machines in the United States.

Cardiomedics Inc.
(provides CardiAssist™ External CounterPulsation)
18872 Bardeen Avenue
Irvine, California 92612
Telephone Number 1-888-849-0200 or 1-949-863-2500
Fax 1-949-474-2274
www.cardiomedics.com

Vasomedical Inc. (Provides EECP®)
180 Linden Avenue
Westbury, New York 11590
Telephone Number 1-800-455-3327 or 1-516-997-4600
Fax 1-516-997-6971
www.eecp.com

The following medical institutions and physicians offer **External CounterPulsation** as described in this book.

Alabama
The Kirklin Clinic
4th Floor - Cardiology Clinic,
2000 6th Avenue
Birmingham, AL 35294
(205) 934-9999

The Heart Center
1215 7th Street
Decatur, AL 35601
(256) 351-0688

Heart Health Center
Eliza Coffee Medical Center
Florence, AL 35631
(256) 768-9646

The Heart Center, P.C.
930 Franklin Avenue
Huntsville, AL 35801
(256) 532-1415
(256) 539-4080

Arizona
Northern Arizona Heart Institute
1753 Airway, Suite B
Kingman, AZ 86401
(520) 757-4359
(520) 697-6200

Montana Cardiology
451 E. 4th Place
Mesa, AZ 85203
(480) 668-5000

HeartGen Centers
10304 N. Hayden Road S-3
Scottsdale, AZ 85258
(480) 368-9616

Arizona Heart Institute
13188 N. 103rd Drive # 301
Sun City, AZ 85351
(623) 933-0557

Dr. Alexander Cadoux
6884 E. Sunrise Dr. Suite 150
Tucson, AZ 85750
(520) 529-9668

Tucson Heart Group
4892 North Stone
Tucson, AZ 85704
(520) 696-4780

Desert Cardiology of Tucson
6367 E. Tanque Verde Rd., Suite 100
Tucson, AZ 85715
(520) 886-3432

Yuma Heart Institute
1773 W. 24th Street
Yuma, AZ 85364
(520) 344-8748

Arkansas
Associates Cardiology
303 E. Matthews
Jonesboro, AR 72401
(870) 935-6729

Cardiology & Medicine Clinic, PA
5315 W. 12th Street
Little Rock, AR 72204
(501) 664-0941

Arkansas Heart
11001 Hermitage Road
Little Rock, AR 72211
(501) 221-2233

Baptist Medical Center
9601 Interstate 630 Exit 7
Little Rock, AR 72205-7299
(501) 202-1422
(501) 221-1422

Heartcare Clinic of Arkansas, P.A.
Doctors Park, 9600 Lile Drive,
Suite 330
Little Rock, AR 72205
(501) 221-7272

Central Arkansas Cardiology
4000 Richards Road
North Little Rock, AR 72117
(501) 758-3999

California
Cardiac Renewal Centers
1716 W. Medical Center Drive
Anaheim, CA 92801
(714) 776-8060

Beverly Hills Counterpulsation Medical
Group, Inc.
125 N. Robertson Blvd.
Beverly Hills, CA 90211
(310) 360-1697

Dr. Bijan Pourat
125 North Robertson Blvd
Beverly Hills, CA 90211
(310) 550-8000

California Diagnostic Center
5400 Balboa Bovd, Suite 122
Encino, CA 91316
(818) 528-2033

Cardiac Renewal Centers
5363 Balboa Avenue #333
Encino, CA 91316
(310) 459-7933

Orange County Cardio
17150 Euclid Street, #306
Fountain Valley, CA 92708
(714) 751-0995
(714) 540-8078

Cardiac Renewal Centers
410 W. Arden Avenue #101
Glendale, CA 91203
(818) 247-7447
(818) 502-6860

Saddleback Hospital
24451 Health Center Dr.
Laguna Hills, CA 92653
(949) 452-7861

Cardiac Renewal Centers
24953 Paseo De Valencia, Suite 6-C
Laguna Hills, CA 92653
(949) 951-4681

Scripps Center for Integrative Medicine
10666 North Torrey Pines Rd,
2nd Fl, Rm. 2011
La Jolla, CA 92037-1092
(858) 554-8751
(858) 554-3300

Cardiac Renewal Centers
500 S. Sepulveda Blvd, Suite 100
Los Angeles, CA 90049
(310) 278-3400
(310) 476-4435

Whitaker Wellness EECP® Center
4321 Birch Street, #3
Newport Beach, CA 92660
(949) 851-1550

Dr. David Steenblock
The Health Restoration Center
26381 Crown Valley Parkway,
Suite 130
Mission Viejo, CA 92691
(949) 367-8870

Dr. Gary Willard
41011 California Oaks Rd., Suite 103
Murrieta, CA 92562
(888) 767-5677

Cardiac Renewal Centers
3998 Vista Way, Suite C-108
Oceanside, CA 92056
(310) 459-7933

Orange County Heart Institute
1140 West La Veta, Suite 640
Orange, CA 92868
(714) 564-3300

Cardiac Renewal Centers
72-880 Fred Warring Road,
Suites D18 & D19
Palm Desert, CA 92260
(310) 459-7933

Cardiac Renewal Centers
301 So. Fairoaks, Suite 207
Pasadena, CA 91105
(626) 229-9905

UCSD Medical Center
200 West Arbor Drive
San Diego, CA 92103-8411
(619) 543-3975

Cardiac Renewal Centers
7625 Mesa College Drive,
Suite 111
San Diego, CA 92111
(310) 459-7933

Ocean View Medical Group
1700 Ocean Avenue
Santa Monica, CA 90401
(310) 899-4000

University of California, San Francisco
Mt. Zion Med. Ctr., 1600 Divisadero
St. Rm. A219
San Francisco, CA 94115-1609
(415) 885-3636

Willard Wellness
40963 Winchester Road
Temecula, CA 92591
(909) 296-5575

Colorado
Dr George Juetersonke
3525 American Drive
Colorado Springs CO 80917
(719) 597-6075

Pikes Peak Cardiology
1625 Medical Center Point, Suite 280
Colorado Springs, CO 80907
(719) 444-3774

Western Cardiology Associates
1601 East 19th Avenue, Suite 5100
Denver, CO 80218
(303) 839-7100

South Denver Cardiology Associates
2535 S. Downing Street, Suite 130
Denver, CO 80210-5848
(303) 744-1065

Kaiser Permanente of Denver
2045 Franklin Street
Denver, CO 80205
(303) 861-3402

Parkview Medical Center
400 West 16th Street
Pueblo, CO 81003
(719) 584-4461
(719) 564-5446

Connecticut
Griffin Hospital
130 Division Street
Derby, CT 06418
(203) 732-7455
(203) 732-7427

Cardiology Associates of Fairfield
County, PC
40 Cross Street, Suite 200
Norwalk, CT 06851
(203) 845-2160

Florida
JFK Medical Center
5301 S. Congress Ave, Card. Rehab,
Rothman 3rd Fl.
Atlantis, FL 33462
(561) 478-1104
(561) 642-3610

Dr. Joseph Shalit
194 Redstone Avenue
Crestview, FL 32539
(850) 682-1022

Shands Hospital
1600 W. Archer Road
Gainesville, FL 32610
(352) 395-0457

James B. DeStephens, MD
2341 N.W. 41st St, Suite B
Gainesville, FL 32606
(352) 371-1804

Neurology & Cardiology Associates
5124 Hollywood Blvd.
Hollywood, FL 33021-2829
(954) 962-2778

South Broward Cardiology
1150 N. 35th Ave Suite 600/605
Hollywood, FL 33021
(954) 983-9182

HealthSouth Rehabilitation
Hospital of Largo
901 N. Clearwater-Largo Road
Largo, FL 33770
(727) 441-8663

Leesburg Heart Group, P.A.
511 Medical Plaza Drive, Suite 101
Leesburg, FL 34748
(352) 728-6808

Demitri C. Pyrros, MD, PA
2825 No State Road 7, Suite 205
Margate, FL 33063
(954) 969-3601

Brevard Cardiology
150 Sykes Creek Parkway # 300
Merritt Island, FL 32953
(321) 452-3811

Osler Medical
930 South Harbor City Blvd.
Melbourne, FL 32901
(321) 725-5050

South Florida Cardiology Associates
11760 Bird Road, Suite 622
Miami, FL 33175
(305) 221-6161

Mt Sinai Medical Center
4300 Alton Road, Suite 207A
Miami Beach, FL 31140
(305) 674-2260

Rodolpho Dumenigo, MD
1423 Alton Road
Miami Beach, FL 33139
(305) 534-0076

Heart Life Cardiac Regenerating Center
2630 NE 203 Street #106
Miami, FL 33180
(305) 935-0168

Miami Heart Institute & Medical
Center
4701 North Meridian Avenue
Miami Beach, FL 33140
(305) 673-0601
(305) 672-1111

South Florida Cardiology Associates
4701 N. Meridan Avenue, Suite 100,
Tower Bldg.
Miami Beach, FL 33140
(305) 672-9989

Lake Cardiology
250 E. 4th Avenue
Mount Dora, FL 32757-5536
(352) 735-1400

Cardiovascular Interventions, P.A.
1900 North Mills Avenue # 3
Orlando, FL 32803
(407) 894-4880

Orlando Heart Center
60 West Gore Street
Orlando, FL 32806
(407) 650-1300

South Florida Cardiology Associates
1601 N. Palm Avenue, Suite 101
Pembroke Pines, FL 33026
(954) 432-1511

Heart & Vascular Institute
3231 McMullen Booth Rd # 102
Safety Harbor, FL 34695
(727) 724-8611

Heart and Vascular Center of Florida
1540 S. Tamiami Trail, 1st Floor
Sarasota, FL 34239
(941) 365-0433

Heart Institute of St. Petersburg
603 7th Street South, # 400
St. Petersburg, FL 33701
(727) 329-1607

Dr. Neil Ahner
705 North Federal Hwy.
Stuart, FL 34994
(561) 692-9200

Stuart Cardiology Group
1001 SE Montery Commons Blvd
Stuart, FL 34994
(561) 286-9400

Palms Heart Center
1501 S. Pinellas Ave., #G
Tarpon Springs, FL 34689
(727) 937-3188

Tarpon Center for Angina Therapy
1501 S. Pinellas Avenue, Suite G
Tarpon Springs, FL 34689
(727) 787-4788
(727) 937 3188

Cardiology & Medicine
Associates, Inc.
3715 Seventh Terrace
Vero Beach, FL 32960
(561) 770-2664

EECP® Heart Center of Vero Beach
777 37th Street, Suite A103
Vero Beach, FL 32960
(561) 569-2710

Georgia
Cardiac Disease Specialist, P.C.
95 Collier Road, NW, Suite 2035
Atlanta, GA 30309
(404) 355-9815

Perennia Heart Centers
P.O. Box 920443
Norcross, GA 300100443
(770) 300-0567

McIntosh Clinic
119 W. Hill Street
Thomasville, GA 31792
(912) 225-1900

Illinois
North Surburban Cardiology Group
1614 W. Central Road, Suite 107
Arlington Heights, IL 60005
(847) 866-6600

Northwest Heart Specialists, SC
1632 W. Central Road
Arlington Heights, IL 60005
(847) 253-8050

St. Francis Hospital
355 Ridge Avenue
Evanston, IL 60202
(847) 864-4370
(847) 316-4150

Dr. Ted Calinog
17850 Kedzie Avenue, Suite 3600
Hazel Crest, IL 60429
(708) 799-9299

Edward Cardiovascular Institute
120 Spalding Drive
Naperville, IL 60540
(630) 527-2741

Christ Hospital and Medical Center
4440 West 95th Street
Oak Lawn, IL 60453
(708) 346-4089
(708) 425-8000

Quincy Cardiac Rehabilitation Center
1005 Broadway
Quincy, IL 62305
(217) 222-6550

Rockford Memorial Hospital
2400 North Rockton Avenue
Rockford, IL 61103
(815) 971-2000
(815) 971-6759

Indiana
Ohio Valley Heart Care
1400 Professional Blvd.
Evansville, IN 47714
(812) 473-2642

The Heart Group
415 West Columbia Street
Evansville, IN 47710
(800) 432-7868

Indiana Cardiac and Vascular
Consultants
1340 E County Line Road, Suite R
Indianapolis, IN 46227
(317) 887-7067

HeartGen Centers
College Park No. 9517 Valparaiso Ct.
Indianapolis, IN 46268
(317) 876-5485

Midwest Internists, P.C.
428 South Main
Lynn, IN 47355
(765) 874-2411

Marion General Hospital
441 Wabash Avenue
Marion, IN 46952
(765) 664-1201
(765) 662-4056

Iowa
St. Luke's Methodist Hospital
1026 A Avenue NE
Cedar Rapids, IA 52406
(319) 369-7211

Mason City Clinic
250 S. Crescent Drive
Mason City, IA 50401
(641) 422-6730

St. Lukes Regional Medical Center
2720 Stone Park Blvd.
Sioux City, IA 51104
(712) 279-3881

Kansas
Cardiology Services
7301 East Frontage Road, Suite 200
Shawnee Mission, KS 66204
(913) 722-0080

EECP® Clinic at Cotton O'Neil
Heart Center
929 Mulvane
Topeka, KS 66604
(785) 270-4125

Louisiana
Heart & Vascular Clinic
101 East Fairway, #206A
Covington, LA 70433
(504) 892-9233

Cardiovascular Institute
4212 W. Congress, Suite 2100
Lafayette, LA 70506
(337) 988-1585

Lester L. Ducote Jr. MD
1211 Coolidge Blvd. Suite 400
Layfayette, LA 70503
(337) 234-3278

Middleton-Cook Medical Corporation
2620 Jena Street
New Orleans, LA 70115
(504) 894-1234

Ochsner Foundation Hospital
1516 Jefferson Highway
New Orleans, LA 70121
(504) 842-3925
(504) 842-3630

Maine
Central Maine Medical Center
300 Main Street
Lewiston, ME 04240
(207) 795-6622

C. V. Diagnostic, Inc
244 Kennedy Memorial Drive
Waterville, ME 04901
(207) 861-5646

Maryland
M. S. Shariff, MD
105 Aurora Street
Cambridge, MD 21513
(410) 901-2221

Howard County General Hospital
A member of Johns Hopkins Medicine
5755 Cedar Lane
Columbia, MD 21044
(410) 461-8100
(410) 740-7890

Beals & Associates
9101 Cherry Lane, Suite 205
Laurel, MD 20708
(301) 490-9914

Adventist Cardiopulmonary Rehab
9715 Medical Center Drive, Suite 130
Rockville, MD 20850
(301) 670-3000
(301) 279-6662

Massachusetts
Cardiovascular Specialists
100 Ter Heun Drive
Falmouth, MA 02540
(508) 540-0604

Path to Health
83 Cambridge Street
Burlington, MA 01803
(781) 221-6996

Michigan
West Michigan Heart
3310 Eagle Park Drive N.E Suite 1002
Grand Rapids, MI 49525
(616) 454-5551

Borgess Medical Center
3025 Gull Road
Kalamazoo, MI 49048
(616) 552-2281

Lansing Cardiovascular
2395 Jolly Road #145
Okemos, MI 48864
(517) 349-3303

Michigan Heart Group
4600 Investment Dr., Suite 200
Troy, MI 48098
(248) 267-5050

Minnesota
Minnesota Heart Clinic
6545 France Ave. South, Suite 150
Edina, MN 55435
(612) 915-2421

Hennepin County Medical Center
701 Park Avenue South
Minneapolis, MN 55415
(612) 347-2875
(612) 347-3704

Paynesville Area Health Sytem
200 First Street West
Paynesville, MN 56362
(320) 243-3767

Mayo Clinic
200 1st Street, SW
Rochester, MN 55905
(507) 255-6092
(507) 255-5891

Mississippi
Cardiovascular Associates, PA
501 Marshall Street
Jackson, MS 39202
(601) 969-2860

Missouri
Missouri Heart Center
Broadway Medical Plaza II, 1605 E.
Broadway, Suite 300
Columbia, MO 65201
(573) 256-3021
(573) 256-3088

Hattiesburg Clinic
415 South 28th Aveue
Hattiesburg, MS 39401
(601) 268-5800

Independence Cardiology
1515 W. Truman Road, Suite 602
Independence, MO 64050
(816) 461-6837

Freeman Health System
1102 West 32nd Street
Joplin, MO 64804
(417) 782-3000

Heart Care and Surgical Associates
2817 McClelland Blvd.
Joplin, MO 64804
(417) 627-8500
(800) 937-3710

St. John's Cardiovascular Specialists
1900 S. National, Suite 3600
Springfield, MO 65804
(417) 841-3911

St. Louis Heart & Vascular
11155 Dunn Road # 304E
St. Louis, MO 63136
(314) 741-0911

Nebraska
Nebraska Heart Institute
1500 South 48th Street, Suite 800
Lincoln, NE 68506
(402) 489-6555

Mary Lanning Hospital
715 North St. Joseph Avenue
Hastings, NE 60901
(402) 461-5256

Consultants in Cardiology
Doctors Building 301S. Tower, 4239
Farnam St.
Omaha, NE 68131
(402) 552-2770

New Hampshire
Elliot Hospital
One Elliot Way
Manchester, NH 03103
(603) 669-5300

Nevada
ECP Heart Centres
3150 N. Tenaya Way, Suite 460
Las Vegas, NV 89128
(702) 480-0356

Heart Institute of Nevada
1090 East Desert Inn Road, Suite 100
Las Vegas, NV 89109
(702) 731-0088

New Jersey
Our Lady of Lourdes
1600 Haddon Ave.
Camden, NJ 08103
(856) 757-3500

Monmouth Cardiology Associates
222 Schanck Road
Freehold, NJ 07728
(732) 431-1332

The Heart-Lung Center
297 Lafayette Avenue
Hawthorne, NJ 075061919
(973) 423-9388

Pavonia Medical
600 Pavonia Avenue
Jersey City, NJ 07306
(201) 216-3060

Heart & Vascular Institute of
New Jersey
111 Madison Avenue, 4th Floor
Morristown, NJ 07960
(973) 656-0555

The Cardiology Group, P.A.
Heart Center
2051 Briggs Road
Mt. Laurel, NJ 08054
(856) 234-3332

University of Medicine & Dentistry of
NJ, University Hospital
150 Bergen Street, Rm I-246
Newark, NJ 07103
(973) 972-4731
(973) 972-5742

Cardiology Associates
28-11 Kennedy Blvd.
North Bergen, NJ 07047
(201) 865-8553

Cardiac Associates of No. Jersey, PA
43 Yawpo Avenue
Oakland, NJ 07436
(201) 337-0066

ECP Heart Center of New Jersey
42 Throckmorton Avenue
Old Bridge, NJ 08857
(732) 679-7972

Cardiology Associates of Paterson
606 Broadway
Paterson, NJ 07514
(973) 278-8818

Preventive Health
555 Shrewsbury Avenue
Shrewsbury, NJ 07702
(732) 389-6455

Central New Jersey Cardiology
1511 Park Avenue, Suite 2
South Plainfield, NJ 07080
(908) 756-4438

Mid-Atlantic Cardiology
211 Mountain Avenue
Springfield, NJ 07081
(973) 467-0005

Cardiology Consultants of
North Jersey
516 Hamburg Tpke
Wayne, NJ 07470
(973) 942-1141

Cardiology Associates
1031 McBride Avenue., Suite B209
West Paterson, NJ 07424
(973) 256-5667
(973) 256-1179

New York
Albany Assoc in Cardiology
2 Palisades Drive
Albany, NY 12205
(518) 458-2000

Robert Potenza, MD, PC
3250 Westchester Avenue
Bronx, NY 10461
(718) 597-9595

Arden Corp
1335 Ocean Parkway
Brooklyn, NY 11230
(718) 236-6264

Cardiology Associates of Brooklyn
848 49th Street
Brooklyn, NY 11219
(718) 283-7948

Professional Medical Arts
1170 Brighton Beach Ave
Brooklyn, NY 11235
(718) 769-1010

Cardiology Associates
40-37 81st Street
Elmhurst, NY 11373
(718) 507-6720

Jamaica Hospital Medical Center
8900 Van Wyck Expressway
Jamaica, NY 11418
(718) 206-7100

Cardiology Associates, P.C.
30 Harrison Street, #250
Johnson City, NY 13790
(607) 770-8600

Long Beach Medical Center
455 East Bay Drive
Long Beach, NY 115612300
(516) 432-2004

Long Island Cardiology & Internal
Medicine
510 Hicksville Road
Massapequa, NY 11758
(516) 795-1500

EECP® of Westchester
105 South Bedford Road
Mount Kisco, NY 10549
(914) 666-2668

Heart Associates of the Finger Lakes
201 Frey Street
Newark, NY 14153
(315) 331-4344

Comprehensive Medical Evaluation
451 Park Avenue
New York, NY 10016
(212) 779-0202

Atkins Center
152 East 55th Street
New York, NY 10022
(212) 758-2110

Beth Israel Medical Center
Dazian Pavillion - 330 East 17th Street
New York, NY 10003
(212) 420-4560
(212) 420-2357

Angina Treatment Centers
1085 Park Avenue
New York, NY 10128
(212) 369-3080
(212) 369-2905

United Hospital Medical Center
406 Boston Post Road
Port Chester, NY 10573
(914) 946-3388

Dr. Mathew Theckedath
1445 Portland Ave, Suite 208
Rochester, NY 14621
(716) 338-2322

George Shapiro, MD, PC
700 White Plains Road
Scarsdale, NY 10583
(914) 472-1900

Staten Island Heart EECP®
1870 Richmond Road
Staten Island, NY 10306
(718) 351-3111

University Medical Center Stony Brook
Cardiology Division, Room T-17-020
Stony Brook, NY 117948171
(631) 444-8420
(631) 444-8114

Dr. Michael Schachter
2 Executive Blvd., Suite 202
Suffern, NY 10901
(914) 368-4700

New York Heart Center
1000 E Genesee Street, #300
Syracuse, NY 13210
(315) 471-1044

EECP® of Nassau
300 Franklin Avenue
Valley Stream, NY 11580
(516) 872-8280

Cardiovascular Wellness Center
1600 Stewart Avenue
Westbury, NY 11590
(516) 222-2288

Health Enhancement
955 Yonkers Avenue
Yonkers, NY 10704
(914) 237-5592

North Carolina
Duke Clinic
#2L, Room 2229, Trent Drive
Durham, NC 27710
(919) 684-5295

Integrative Cardiology Assoc.
4140 Mendenhall Oaks Pkwy #101
High Point, NC 27265
(336) 841-1259

Wake Heart Associates
4325 Lake Boone Trail, Suite 300
Raleigh, NC 27607
(919) 231-8253
(919) 420-1347

Ohio
Cleveland Clinic
9500 Euclid Ave. Department of
Cardiology-F25
Cleveland, OH 44106
(216) 444-6712
(219) 444-8128

Preventative Medicine Group
24700 Center Ridge Road, Suite 317
Cleveland, OH 44145
(440) 835-0104

EECP® Center of The Ohio Heart
2123 Auburn Avenue, Suite 231
Cincinnati, OH 45219
(513) 287-8500
(513) 287-8518

Cardiovascular Research Institute, Inc.
300 E. Town Street, Suite 1600
Columbus, OH 43215
(614) 324-9090

EECP® Center of Northwest Ohio
4607 Sylvania Avenue, Suite 200
Toledo, OH 43623
(419) 882-9620
(419) 882-9625

Associates in Cardiovascular Medicine
495 Cooper Road, Suite 427
Westerville, OH 43081
(614) 575-2811

St. John West Shore Hospital
29000 Center Ridge Road
Westlake, OH 44145
(440) 323-0882

Oklahoma
Cardiovascular Clinic (Div. of Plaza
Medical Group PC)
3433 Northwest 56th Street
Oklahoma City, OK 73112
(405) 947-3341

Oklahoma Cardiovascular Associates
1110 N. Classen Blvd
Oklahoma City, OK 73102
(405) 271-1350

Oregon
Heart Centers of America, LLC
Physicians Office Bldg .
2222 NW Lovejoy St, Suite 512
Portland, OR 97210
(503) 222-0262

Pennsylvania
The Heart Care Group, PC
Jaindl Family Pavilion, Suite 500 -
1202 South Cedar Crest Blvd.
Allentown, PA 18103
(610) 437-5505

Brookville Hospital
100 Hospital Road
Brookville, PA 15825
(814) 849-4442

Consultants in Cardiology, Inc.
311 W. 24th Street, Suite 401
Erie, PA 16502
(814) 453-7767

Cardiac Renewal East
1740 South Street
Philadelphia, PA 19146
(215) 772-9800

EECP® Center of Pittsburgh
1350 Locust Avenue
Pittsburgh, PA 15219
(412) 562-3292

University of Pittsburgh Medical
Center
200 Lothrop St., 6F-Rm. 685,
Cardiology Out-Patient
Pittsburgh, PA 152132582
(412) 647-6136
(412) 647-0280

Century Cardiac Care Incorporated
1668 Lincoln Way
White Oak, PA 15131
(412) 664-4124

Apple Hill Medical Center
25 Monument Road, Suite 199,
Entrance C
York, PA 17403
(717) 741-4690

Puerto Rico
Cardiologia Invasiva e Interventional
Calie Guadalype Final, Antiguo
Hospital
San Lucas, Ponce, Puerto Rico 00731

South Carolina
South Carolina Heart Center
2001 Laurel Street
Columbia, SC 29204
(803) 765-9044
(803) 376-8026

Upstate Cardiology
1005 Grove Road
Greenville, SC 29605
(864) 235-7665

South Dakota
Sioux Valley Hospital
1100 South Euclid Avenue
Sioux Falls, SD 57105
(605) 357-2929

Avera McKennan Hospital
800 E. 21st Street
Sioux Falls, SD 57105
(605) 357-1340

Tennessee
Regional Cardiology Consultants
111 Stonebridge Avenue
Jackson, TN 38305
(901) 664-4446

Knoxville Cardiovascular Group
Professional Office Bldg. 2 Suite 260 -
1932 Alcoa Highway
Knoxville, TN 37920
(865) 544-2800

East Tennessee Heart Consultants, PC
Suite 300, Baptist Medical Tower, 101
Blount Avenue
Knoxville, TN 37920
(865) 673-9656

Memphis Heart Alliance
5959 Park Avenue
Memphis, TN 38119
(901) 765-1740

Cardiovascular Physicians of Memphis
Suite 100, 4901 Raleigh Common
Drive
Memphis, TN 38128
(901) 371-9040

Stephen Humble, MD
341 Wallace Road, Suite A
Nashville, TN 37211
(615) 834-7744

Texas
Heartplace
515 W. Mayfield, Suite 201
Arlington, TX 76014
(817) 468-2028

BCS Heart, LLP
1605 Rock Prairie Road, #310
College Station, TX 77845
(979) 764-1474

Cardiology Associates of Corpus
Christi
1521 South Staples
Corpus Christi, TX 78404
(361) 888-8261

Advanced Heartcare
8230 Walnut Hill Lane, Suite 620
Dallas, TX 75231
(214) 739-0404

The Dallas Heart Group
7777 Forest Lane, S 202
Dallas, TX 75230
(972) 566-7733

Children's Medical Center
1935 Motor Street
Dallas, TX 75235
(214) 456-8738

Heartplace
411 North Washington # 2200
Dallas, TX 75246
(800) 841-0422

Advanced Heartcare
609 Medical Center Drive, Suite 2100
Decatur, TX 76234
(940) 627-0044

El Paso Heart Clinic
1300 Murchison, Suite 200
El Paso, TX 79902
(915) 532-4542

Dr. Whitaker
210 E Elizabeth
Jefferson, TX 75657
(800) 232-6234
(903) 665-7781

E.C.P. of South Texas
4762 Kingfisher Drive
Houston, TX 77035
(713) 721-6676
(713) 721-0190

Heart Associates of Texas
4126 Southwest Freeway, Suite 200
Houston, TX 77027
(713) 622-4505

St. Lukes Episcopal Hospital
6624 Fannin, Medical Tower 11thFloor
Cardiology
Houston, TX 77030
(713) 791-8500

Houston Assoc of Cardiovascular
Medicine
4126 SW Freeway
Houston, TX 77027
(713) 599-1144

The Heart Center at Heart Place
Hospital
25 Village Circle
Midland, TX 79701
(915) 683-2455

Advanced Heartcare
1025 DeShong
Paris, TX 75462
(888) 322-7268

Southeast Houston Cardiology
4004 Woodlawn Avenue
Pasadena, TX 77504
(713) 946-7588

Johnson Medical Associates
317 Dal-Rich Village
Richardson TX 75080
(972) 479-0400
(800) 807-7555

Texas Cardiovascular
5702 Rowlett Road # 210
Rowlett, TX 75088
(972) 412-3583

Houston Heart & Vascular Associates
2205 Williams Trace Blvd.
Sugar Land, TX 77478
(281) 277-3939

Utah
Murray Health Center
2046 E. Murray Holladay Rd., Suite
100
Salt Lake City, UT 84117
(801) 277-5000

Red Cliff Nutritional Center
321 North Mall Drive #L103
St. George, UT 84790
(435) 674-3500

Central Utah Medical Clinic,
Cardiology Department
1055 North 500
West Provo, UT 84604
(801) 373-4366

Vermont
Integrative Cardiology
8 Commons Street
Rutland, VT 05701
(802) 775-0100

Virginia
University of Virginia
2955 Ivy Rd, Suite 211 - Northridge
Charlottesville, VA 22903
(804) 924-2420
(804) 924-2999

EECP® Center of Northern Virginia
8316 Arlington Blvd. Suite 500
Fairfax, VA 22031
(703) 641-9161

Riverside Regional Medical Center
500 J. Clyde Morris Blvd
Newport News, VA 23601
(757) 594-2074

Cardiovascular Associates of Virginia,
P. C.
681 Hioaks Road, Suite H
Richmond, VA 23225
(804) 323-1804

West Virginia
Ruby Memorial Hospital
Medical Center Drive
Morgantown, WV 265068003
(304) 293-4096
(304) 598-4248

Wisconsin
Cardiovascular Associates of Northern
Wisconsin
520 North 28th Avenue
Wausau, WI 64401
(715) 847-2611

Useful Web Sites

Dr. Juetersonke's web site
www.drjlifepulse.com

External CounterPulsation Web Sites
Cardiomedics - www.cardiomedics.com
Vasomedical - www.eecp.com

University of California at San Francisco
http://cardio.ucsf.edu/clinical/eecp/
Mayo Clinic
http://mayohealth.org/mayo/0005/htm/eecp.htm

Laboratories for Cholesterol Testing
Berkeley - www.berkeleyheartlab.com
Great Smokies Diagnostics - www.gsdl.com./index.shtml
Mayo Clinic - www.mayo.edu/pathlab/pathmain.htm
Nichols Institute Diagnostics - www.nicholsdiag.com/index.html
Antibody Assay Laboratory - www.antibodyassay.com/

Ultrafast CT Electron Beam Tomography
www.coloradoheart.com
www.heartinfo.com/schem2.html

General Information Sites
American Heart Association - www.americanheart.org
Dr. Dean Edell - www.healthcentral.com
Dr. Koop's web site - www.drkoop.com

Finance Companies
Hillside Patient Financing - www.affordablepayments.com
Unicorn financial - www.howtopayforit.com

George J. Juetersonke D.O., is a native of Illinois. He studied medicine at Midwestern University, Chicago College of Osteopathic Medicine, is Board Certified in Family Practice and has been actively practicing medicine as a physician for 20 years. For five years he served on the full time medical faculty of The University of North Texas Health Science Center were he was an Assistant Professor in the Department of Preventive Medicine. He continues to hold a faculty appointment as Clinical Assistant Professor at The University of North Texas Health Science Center in Fort Worth.

Medical students and residents are frequently found in Dr. Juetersonke's office where they often spend a month studying the clinical aspects of preventive medicine. Much of the time Dr. Juetersonke can be found lecturing to physicians at meetings across the country as well as to the general public. Dr. Juetersonke has a special interest in Syndrome X (Coronary artery disease, Hypertension, Adult onset diabetes, Obesity, and Stroke).

Dr. Juetersonke is a member of the American Osteopathic Association, Colorado Society of Osteopathic Medicine, Colorado Springs Osteopathic Medical Foundation, El Paso County Medical Society, member of the board of Foundation for Environmental Research in Colorado, and former senior editor for AAEM Medical Digest.

Visit Dr. Juetersonke at his website:
www.drjlifepulse.com

Dr. Juetersonke regularly travels the United States giving numerous lectures on many subjects including heart disease. If you would like to know where you can see Dr. Juetersonke in person or would like to have him speak to your group contact his office at:

Dr. Juetersonke
3525 American Drive
Colorado Springs CO 80917
Telephone 719-597-6075

Or visit the website.

Need information? Call or write to the above address.